No More
Fatigue

Also by Jack Challem

The Inflammation Syndrome
Stop Prediabetes Now
The Food-Mood Solution
Feed Your Genes Right
Syndrome X

No More Fatigue

Why You're So Tired and What You Can Do about It

JACK CHALLEM

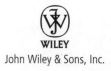

WILEY

John Wiley & Sons, Inc.

Published by John Wiley & Sons, Inc., Hoboken, New Jersey
Published simultaneously in Canada

Design by Forty-Five Degree Design LLC

Library of Congress Cataloging-in-Publication Data:
Challem, Jack.
  No more fatigue : why you're so tired and what you can do about it /
Jack Challem.
      p. cm.
   Includes bibliographical references and index.
   ISBN 978-0-470-52545-6 (cloth); ISBN 978-0-470-93080-9 (ebk.); ISBN 978-0-470-93082-3 (ebk.); ISBN 978-0-470-93083-0 (ebk.)
1. Fatigue–Popular works. 2. Chronic fatigue syndrome–Popular
works. I. Title.
RB150.F37C42 2011
616'.0478–dc22
                                              2010046364

Printed in the United States of America

10 9 8 7 6 5 4 3 2 1

For all the special people in my life

Contents

Foreword

Health is having the reserve to do what you want to do
and need to do with energy and enthusiasm.

Hugh Riordan, M.D.
1932–2005

My medical mentor got it right: health and energy go hand in hand. When personal energy reserves run low, it becomes much more difficult to satisfy basic human needs. Frustration, depression, and a pervasive attitude of defeat creep into every aspect of your life. Overwhelming fatigue emerges as the harbinger of ill health and disease.

Many studies have shown that fatigue is the chief reason why people see their doctors. I estimate that one of every two patients I see complains of fatigue. Sometimes the cause is obvious, such as when a woman is trying to do too much between home and work. For men, fatigue is often a consequence of poor eating habits or disturbed sleep. The underlying causes can range from an age-related hormonal imbalance to an unsuspected emerging illness, such as prediabetes, depression, or cancer. Lifestyle issues are almost always a factor, too.

When I talk with patients about the origins of their fatigue, I wonder what became of the boundless energy we had as children. What happened to that endless reserve of energy and enthusiasm that fueled our creative play? The truth is, sad to say, that the nearly inevitable stresses of our crazy world wear us down and rob us of vital life energy.

Everything in life comes back to energy. Physical energy runs our cars and heats our homes. Emotional energy propels us into the relationships that give meaning to our lives. Mental energy allows us to envision goals and then strive to achieve them. Spiritual energy, though invisible and immeasurable, underlies our will to live and love. Buckminster Fuller went so far as to state that 90 percent of what it means to be human is invisible. He was talking about energy.

Not surprisingly, the need for energy is also a truism in biology and biochemistry. All forms of life depend on food for growth, health, and energy. When we (and all of those other life forms) consume food, some of the nutrients are broken down to create energy. As biological creatures, we depend on these biochemical processes to properly fuel our cells and maintain our organ functions. High-quality functioning depends on high-quality foods and fuels.

Yet faced with day-to-day stresses and dwindling energy reserves, we often turn to quick fixes. Coffee and other caffeine-containing beverages are now ubiquitous. So are sugar-rich foods. Soft-drink machines, fast-food drive-thrus, coffee huts, and a whole range of convenience options set us up to become quick-fix addicts. In essence, people end up using caffeine and sugar to self-medicate, to give them more energy. As you might have already noticed, however, there is a point of diminishing returns. These stimulants can interfere with sleep, which we must have to recoup our energy. After a while, most people need a little more caffeine or sugar, then a little more, and then still a little more. The irony is that these uppers can often turn into downers.

Obviously, quick fixes become crutches and are never long-term solutions. People who have become too dependent on coffee and sweets often lead lives that are out of balance. They're like laboratory mice running furiously on an exercise wheel but going nowhere fast. The faster they go, the more tired they feel and the less aware they become of the underlying causes of their declining productivity. More often than not, they'll eventually be diagnosed with a serious illness. Their bodies finally cave in and collapse in some kind of breakdown or health crisis.

Nearly everyone has experienced this kind of burnout at one time or another. That's the nature of modern life. If you're taking the time to read this book, odds are that you're already seeing yourself in these pages. Know this: there are ways to achieve equilibrium, a balance between a well-deserved feeling of temporary fatigue and the energy to enjoy your work and your play.

The long-term solution to fatigue and a lack of energy is actually one you can control—if you take the time to look beyond the quick fixes that really don't work. There are many important reasons for working on your own energy plan. The immediate benefit, of course, is that you'll feel better and have more energy. Down the line, you'll reduce your risk of serious illness, because fatigue can be both an early symptom of festering health problems and a consequence of serious diseases.

During the last ten years or so, Jack Challem and I have become friends and occasional professional collaborators and coauthors. I am continually amazed by his insights in nutrition and medicine, and we often influence each other's thinking about these subjects.

Jack's recent books reflect a blend of his personal and professional journeys. When I first met Jack, his major health complaint was fatigue. The apparent cause was prediabetes, which he soon reversed without any medications. Years later, after a period of unusual stress in his life, he developed symptoms of adrenal burnout, which he again reversed through improvements in his eating habits, the use of certain nutritional supplements, and lifestyle changes. That's why he wrote this book—to share what he has learned with you before a breakdown occurs.

His books also reflect a progression in his thinking from dealing with individual health problems, such as Syndrome X and prediabetes, to a much more holistic and integrative view of health. This book, *No More Fatigue*, provides a wealth of advice for ending fatigue and improving your energy level. To frame his discussion, Jack introduces you to two new and important ways of thinking about fatigue: first, the Fatigue

Syndrome and, second, the five circles (or principal causes) of fatigue that form the syndrome.

This is a fantastic book that I will share with many of my patients. If you're more tired than you think you should be, this book will likely help you as well. I encourage you to read it and change your life for the better. Yes, you can rediscover that youthful joy of life by rebuilding your health reserves "with energy and enthusiasm."

Ron Hunninghake, M.D.

Acknowledgments

Expressing gratitude is good for one's health, so this page is of special importance for my well-being. I learn something from everyone I meet and communicate with, and I must acknowledge all of you who remain unnamed simply because of a lack of space. I have learned from talking with countless physicians and researchers: you have all been kind enough to share some of your precious time and knowledge. I have learned from my clients to whom I coach nutrition; you have motivated me to keep learning so that I can help you and many others.

There are several individuals I would like to name specifically. One is my good friend Ron Hunninghake, M.D., who somehow finds the time for our friendship, despite his family and professional commitments. I must acknowledge the lasting influence of my older brother, Mel, who died many years ago—and whose death happened to chart the course of my professional and personal lives. I must pay homage to two of my teachers, whom I have acknowledged on previous occasions: the late Harold G. Miller, who shaped so much of my creativity when I was still rough around the edges, and Dr. Dewitt Garrett, who catalyzed my interest in nutrition. In the field of nutritional medicine, I also owe much to the late Abram Hoffer, M.D., Ph.D., who was always so gracious with his time and who viewed the worlds of nutrition and medicine from a unique perspective.

There are other people, too, such as those who refined my interest in nutrition and physical activity. I might not have always acknowledged you, but you did help me on my personal path to health, and I keep trying to spread your wisdom. Finally, I would like to thank Tom Miller, my editor at John Wiley & Sons, Inc. This is our sixth book together! I also appreciate the diligence of production editors John Simko and Hope Breeman—and the exceptional line-by-line copyediting by Patricia Waldygo. Thank you also, Jack Scovil, my literary agent.

Introduction

Janet figured that she was a successful supermom. She had two small children in day care and worked a high-pressure job in advertising. Yet even though her husband was helpful, Janet was often stretched while juggling the demands of work, being a parent, and doing her share of grocery shopping and cooking. She thought she could get by on five hours of sleep each night. Then one day, she said, she simply "hit the wall." She was totally wiped out.

Richard's life was one of constant deadlines at a high-tech company. He often had only a cup of coffee and a bagel for breakfast, drank more coffee to keep going through the day, skipped lunch, and then crashed on the sofa after eating dinner. When Richard finally went to bed, he spent much of the night tossing and turning and then woke up very tired in the morning. On Fridays, he usually went out for beer and pizza with his coworkers. Richard often told his TGIF friends that he was completely zonked and brain dead at the end of the week.

Lynn, a middle manager, practically worked 24/7 directing her employees, preparing budgets and expense reports, and fielding e-mails from international customers until late at night and on weekends. After all, it might be midnight here, but it was the middle of the business day at her company's office in Tokyo. Would Lynn ever take a vacation to recharge? Of course not. Now in her forties, Lynn was gaining weight and felt so tired on most days that once she almost had a car accident during her commute home.

With all of the energy-zapping pressures of work and home life, we've developed an odd lexicon to describe how we feel. We're not simply tired or fatigued anymore. We describe ourselves as wiped out, burned out, worn out, wasted, hammered, bushed, drained, whacked, zapped, zonked, run down, or brain dead. I call this persistent state of exhaustion the "Fatigue Syndrome" because it usually involves more than just one cause.

Janet's, Richard's, and Lynn's stories ring so true because their lives remind us of ourselves. These three people have done their best to navigate the pressures of life, but the stresses eventually caught up with them. Their fatigue became almost debilitating. They were still functioning— sort of—doing their work and tackling chores at home. Yet everything in their lives became weighed down by physical and mental fatigue. Were they enjoying life? Were they functioning at their best? They said they were, but you can draw your own conclusions.

What was the cause of their fatigue? Each of them suffered from a primary cause, such as poor dietary habits, hormonal imbalances (for example, low adrenal or thyroid hormones), or inadequate rest. These "causes," however, were actually emblematic of broader issues that formed the Fatigue Syndrome. Only after recognizing and correcting the underlying reasons for their fatigue were Janet, Richard, and Lynn able to regain their energy, vigor, and enthusiasm for life.

According to articles in medical journals and physicians' reports about their patients, one in every four people goes through life feeling perpetually fatigued. The actual number is likely higher. A survey conducted by a company that tracks consumer trends found that one-third of Americans reported having less energy compared with a year earlier.

I've heard people complain about their fatigue in Tucson, Arizona, where I live, and in audiences I have spoken to in Chicago, New York, San Francisco, and many other cities. Like a shock wave that encircled the world, the Fatigue Syndrome is now so common in modern life that it drags down people in Montreal, London, Istanbul, and other cities where I've lectured about nutrition and lifestyle.

I have good news, though. If you're one of the millions of people who muddles through a daily personal energy crisis, you can permanently banish your feelings of fatigue and safely increase your energy level without using any stimulants.

I speak from personal experience, backed up by evidence from the lives of clients I've coached in nutrition and the stories so many other people have told me. I'll start by describing my own two bouts of extreme fatigue.

In the early 1990s, my energy levels were at an all-time low. At that time, my first wife and I were the parents of an infant, and nearly every parent knows how the combined demands of work and raising a small child can suck away every bit of one's energy. In addition to often feeling tired physically, I frequently had difficulty concentrating after eating lunch or dinner.

It took a few years, but I eventually discovered the underlying cause of my fatigue: blood tests showed that my blood sugar was elevated, and I was prediabetic. This is a very common problem, affecting at least 100 million Americans, and fatigue and poor concentration (especially after eating) are common signs of prediabetes. As a health and nutrition writer, I was embarrassed, but that embarrassment gave way to action. Little by little, I revamped my eating habits, took some nutritional supplements to stabilize my blood sugar, and began to exercise. With these changes (and no medications), my blood sugar improved, and I had energy to do all of the things I wanted to in life.

My second brush with serious fatigue, coincidentally, occurred during the early months of writing this book. I had recently gone through a divorce, had helped two friends who were diagnosed with cancer, and was involved in a new romantic relationship. That relationship entailed a lot of very late nights—we often stayed up until three in the morning, talking and laughing on the sofa. Although it was fun, I became sleep deprived and found myself drinking a lot of coffee in the morning and needing afternoon naps. I also noticed that I felt dizzy if I stood up too quickly.

Talk about serendipity! At the time, I was researching and writing the chapter that focused on adrenal exhaustion—another very common cause of fatigue—and I realized that I had many of its symptoms. The dizziness is known medically as orthostatic hypotension: low blood pressure that occurs when one gets up from a chair or a stooped position. I visited Dr. Ron Hunninghake in Wichita, Kansas, and a saliva cortisol test confirmed that my adrenal hormones were at their rock bottom. The solution included taking over-the-counter adrenal extracts, using certain herbs that enhance adrenal hormones, and making a point of going to sleep earlier. A few months later, I was back to normal and all too aware of how fatigue can sneak up on a person.

I have to be upfront with you. If you're hoping to read about a single pill, a super-energy food, or a shot of caffeine that will rev up your energy for five hours or more, I'm sorry. You won't find any quick fixes that really work long term—here or anyplace else, for that matter. A lot of advertisements promise you hours of energy from one stimulant or another, but the truth is that they don't work—or they end up causing an energy crash, the opposite of what you want.

---

quick tip
The Semantics of Fatigue

Certain experts and authors have tried to make a point of distinguishing the differences between fatigue, exhaustion, tiredness, and other terms that describe a significant lack of physical or mental energy. In my opinion, this has often turned into a meaningless "name game." You know that your problem is a lack of energy, and I will use terms such as *fatigued* and *tired* interchangeably in this book.

I believe that your first step should be to ask yourself, "Why do I feel so tired?" When you come up with the most obvious reason, then you have to look just a little deeper to identify the real cause of your fatigue. As you dig into the causes of your fatigue, you will inevitably discover how the Fatigue Syndrome has dragged you down.

I'll give you an example. People often tell me that they are tired because they don't get enough sleep. If feeling tired were only a sleep issue, the solution would be easy—simply go to bed earlier or sleep a little later. Yet many people don't sleep well, and others sleep a full eight hours every night and still wake up feeling tired.

A lack of restful sleep is often related to other problems, such as stress from work, anxiety over personal relationships, drinking too much coffee or alcohol, feeling depressed, having difficulty turning off an active brain, being addicted to late-night e-mailing and texting, hot flashes in women, or prostate enlargement and related urinary problems in men. It might seem simple to treat ongoing sleep problems with a prescription drug, an herb, or an over-the-counter nutritional supplement, but focusing only on the sleep problem ignores the other factors that cause fatigue and lack of sound sleep. Then there are the side effects from medications: in other words, Ambien and Lunesta might put you to sleep, but at what cost? Plus, they don't correct the real reasons why you can't sleep. To improve your sleep, you must identify and then remedy the underlying causes.

Cultivating this type of broader thinking is essential if you want to permanently overcome the Fatigue Syndrome and increase your energy. Some people would describe the approach as holistic or integrative, but this doesn't mean it will be complicated or will take a long time before you see any benefits. To the contrary, even if you follow only some of my recommendations, you will likely have much more energy within a day or two.

What Are the Five Circles of Fatigue?

A syndrome is a cluster of related signs or symptoms that either directly cause or are intertwined with health problems. The idea of the Fatigue Syndrome is built around my concept of the "five circles of fatigue."

These circles represent the most common causes of fatigue and they usually form a cluster and a syndrome. In many people who feel fatigued, one or two of the circles tend to dominate, but the other three circles might also contribute to fatigue.

The Five Circles of Fatigue
1. Stress
2. Poor dietary habits
3. Hormone imbalances
4. Chronic illnesses (and many medications)
5. The aging process

These circles of fatigue usually develop in a sequential way—that is, one circle lays the groundwork for the next one. Often, some of the five circles of fatigue will overlap, and occasionally they might flow in reverse. I'll explain just a little about the five circles here, but I'll go into more detail in chapters 1 through 5.

Stress sets the stage for, and exacerbates, the other four circles of fatigue. It disrupts eating habits, alters hormone levels, increases the risk of serious illness, and accelerates the aging process.

Eating habits are important because nutrients form the foundation of our biochemistry and our hormones. The foods we eat are a major influence on our risk of developing certain diseases (such as obesity, diabetes, heart disease, and cancer) and on the aging process itself. Healthy foods support our bodies' biochemical ability to make energy; unhealthy foods leave us feeling wiped out.

Hormones are strongly influenced by stress and our eating habits. Our adrenal hormones help insulate us from stress, and thyroid hormones play a key role in our bodies' ability to burn food for energy. Long-term stress eventually depletes our adrenal hormones, and by middle age, many women experience a decrease in their thyroid hormone levels. Doctors often fail to diagnose adrenal exhaustion or hypothyroidism because they order the wrong tests or misinterpret vague test results.

Illnesses can be a consequence of stress, poor eating habits, low hormone levels, or all three factors. People with type 2 diabetes, chronic fatigue syndrome, fibromyalgia, cancer, arthritis, and serious heart disease often feel tired a lot of the time. Many medications, such as cholesterol-lowering statins, interfere with normal muscle and liver function and leave people feeling weak and tired.

Aging, a normal process, inevitably affects our energy levels. The first four circles of fatigue can make you age faster—and can leave you feeling older than you really are. Yet many centenarians have more energy than people in their seventies do. Scientists have discovered that certain consequences of aging can be modified.

For Jan, Adrenal Exhaustion Led to Chronic Fatigue Syndrome

Jan was literally one of America's toughest cops. She loved the adrenaline rush of patrolling the streets as a uniformed officer, and even after she rose through the ranks to become a supervisory officer, she still relished being in the middle of the action. Routine weeks were punctuated by episodes of intense heart-pounding stress—chasing suspected criminals, being in shootouts, and dodging bullets. Yet Jan was addicted to the high-intensity thrill of it all.

She often ate on the run, consuming too many fast-food meals and drinking large amounts of coffee to stay sharp. She knew her eating habits could be better, but she simply didn't have the time to cook or eat healthier meals. Then one day her world fell apart. In the middle of a shootout, she collapsed from overwhelming fatigue. The years of chronic stress had caught up with her; she was physically wiped out and had to retire on disability.

Jan's diagnosis was complicated. She was initially diagnosed with chronic fatigue syndrome (CFS), but the CFS was not precipitated by an infection. Her collapse in the field was actually due to adrenal exhaustion. Her body's ability to make adrenal hormones—an important buffer against stress—had worn out, and not even two pots of coffee a day could keep her going any longer.

Finally, under the care of a nutritionally oriented physician, Jan focused on improving her eating habits and taking several natural supplements to enhance her energy levels. Little by little, her health moved back from the brink, and she learned to modulate her activities to avoid another physical collapse. Jan eventually found a satisfying new career, and this time around, she was more mindful of the consequences of stress.

Why This Book Is Different

You may wonder how the fatigue-fighting, energy-enhancing program in *No More Fatigue* is different from advice you might read in other books or on the Web. There are several important differences.

First and foremost, this book addresses the most common causes of fatigue—stress, poor eating habits, low hormone levels, chronic illness and medications, and the aging process—in an integrated fashion. No other book has tackled the Fatigue Syndrome in quite this way, and I provide clear and safe solutions to banish fatigue and naturally enhance and sustain your energy levels.

Second, many authors have ignored the role of low adrenal hormones (adrenal exhaustion or burnout) and low thyroid hormones in fatigue. Often, physicians aren't much help either, because they have difficulty diagnosing borderline cases of adrenal exhaustion or low thyroid activity. Indeed, one clue to adrenal exhaustion is the need to consume large amounts of Starbucks high-caffeine brew daily. (A 16-ounce Starbucks grande-size coffee contains the amount of caffeine found in about ten cans of Coca-Cola or Pepsi!) I'll help you navigate this fuzzy medical area, so that you can take the necessary steps to improve your energy levels.

Third, many approaches to increasing your energy revolve around the use of stimulants in one form or another (such as caffeine), herbs (for example, guarana), or drugs (such as Ritalin). The excessive use of stimulants has undesirable health consequences and, over the long run, also has diminishing benefits. Stimulants push your body in unnatural ways, creating dependencies or addictions, and eventually force you to use larger amounts to maintain your energy levels. That's why so many people feel tired even when they consume five to ten cups of coffee daily. Stimulants also tend to have a yo-yo effect, with energy levels plummeting between "hits."

Third, some energy-boosting ideas focus exclusively on nutritional supplements. I take nutritional supplements, and I believe they can help maximize one's energy, but I recommend them as part of a broader program. Many companies market supplements that claim to be the ultimate solution for everyone's energy problems, yet they ignore all of the other important ways people can boost their energy. Although taking a pill might seem appealing, simple solutions rarely, if ever, provide long-term benefits.

Fourth, some authors have recommended specific diets to improve energy levels. These diets vary, with some being more or less on the right track, and others making absolutely no nutritional or biochemical sense. For example, diets that are very high in carbohydrates tend to decrease energy levels, not increase them. Even the best of these diets focuses too much on foods and not enough on nondietary causes of fatigue. Again, they end up being a partial solution, not a complete one.

Finally, some authors recommend exercise programs to increase energy levels. The problem here is that people who feel tired all of the time can't imagine having enough energy to exercise. Exercise does increase one's energy, but a program of physical activity must begin slowly and be carefully graduated to avoid adding to a person's fatigue.

Many other approaches to the Fatigue Syndrome have a similar undercurrent: they are typically simplistic or narrow, with the basic idea being something like "Drink this liquid, take this pill, eat this food, or lift these weights . . . and your energy levels will miraculously increase." Believe me, I wish things were that simple. If they were that easy, no one would ever feel tired. With millions of people complaining of fatigue, however, it's obvious that either these approaches don't work or people can't stick with them.

In *No More Fatigue,* I provide a more comprehensive, step-by-step approach that can boost and then sustain your energy levels—safely, without pushing your body in harmful ways. My questionnaire on pages 11–14 will help you understand what aspect of your life is primarily responsible for most of your feelings of fatigue.

A lot of what you'll read in this book may surprise you. Here is a foretaste of what you will learn:

- Sugar is not an energy food—it actually makes you more tired.
- Coffee is not an energy drink—and drinking too much will eventually leave you feeling very tired.
- Adrenal exhaustion may be the most common hormone disorder that doctors fail to diagnose.
- Low thyroid hormone levels often overlap with low estrogen levels in women in their forties and fifties, but many doctors seem to miss the connection and overlook a common cause of fatigue.
- Drinking just a tiny bit of caffeine in the late afternoon or evening can ruin a good night's sleep, making people "need" more coffee the next morning to sharpen up.
- The more overweight you are, the more likely it is that you will feel tired, so losing weight will help you feel more energized.
- A large number of common medications, including antidepressants, antihistamines, and cholesterol-lowering drugs, can lower your energy levels.

On the positive side:

- Many foods provide sustained energy, but you probably wouldn't guess which ones. I explain what foods to eat (and to avoid) in chapter 2.
- Do you suffer from adrenal exhaustion or an underactive thyroid gland? I'll help you make a determination in chapter 3.
- You can use safe nutritional supplements to enhance your adrenal function and boost the activity of an underactive thyroid gland. I explain how in chapter 3.

■ Can some nutritional supplements improve your energy without acting as unnatural stimulants? The answer is yes, and I make my recommendations in chapter 6.

■ Exercise can boost your energy levels, but too little or too much can have the opposite effect. I explain how to exercise for energy in chapter 11.

That's only a sampling of the advice you'll find in *No More Fatigue*. The next step is to take the "five circles of fatigue" questionnaire, to learn whether you suffer from the Fatigue Syndrome.

The Fatigue Syndrome Questionnaire

Unfortunately, there is no single medical test to determine the source of your fatigue. Doctors might order a variety of tests, based on their hunches and on what they find in a physical examination. Your answers to the following questions should help you identify some of the causes of your fatigue.

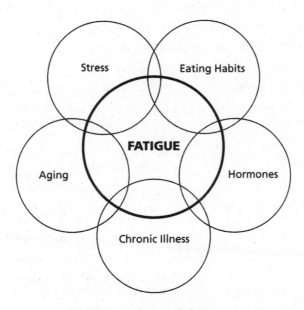

The Five Circles of Fatigue

Stress and Lifestyle

I feel as though there is a lot of stress in my life.	Y/N
I tend to get angry at other people, such as family members, coworkers, and slow drivers.	Y/N
I feel tired when I wake up in the morning.	Y/N
I feel tired much of the time.	Y/N
I feel tired after moderate physical activity, such as a walk, cleaning the house, or mowing the lawn.	Y/N
I find it necessary to sleep late on weekends to catch up on a lack of sleep from the week before.	Y/N
I have difficulty falling asleep or staying asleep because I keep thinking about work or family issues.	Y/N
I am the parent of an infant or a small child.	Y/N
I find that maintaining a personal relationship wears me out.	Y/N
I often fall asleep while watching television.	Y/N
I don't have the time for regular exercise.	Y/N
I work the swing or graveyard shift.	Y/N
I don't have enough downtime.	Y/N
I don't spend much time in the sun or outdoors.	Y/N
I feel "down" or depressed a lot of the time.	Y/N
I worry or have anxiety about a lot of things.	Y/N
Regardless of my sex, I tend to get angry and short-tempered when I'm stressed or don't have enough time to do things.	Y/N

Eating Habits

I need to have coffee, cola, or an energy drink to fully wake up and be alert in the morning.	Y/N
I get a headache when I don't have my coffee (or other caffeinated drink).	Y/N
I have three or more cups of coffee (or other caffeinated drink) each day.	Y/N
I either skip breakfast or eat some type of starchy food, such as bread, cereal, pancakes, or a breakfast bar.	Y/N

I feel tired after lunch or dinner. Y/N

I have two or more alcoholic drinks each day. Y/N

I eat at McDonald's, Burger King, KFC, Taco Bell, or some
other type of fast-food restaurant at least once every week. Y/N

I eat at McDonald's, Burger King, KFC, Taco Bell, or some
other type of fast-food restaurant almost every day. Y/N

I eat a packaged microwave meal at home or at the office
one or more times each week. Y/N

I make a point of eating low-fat foods. Y/N

I tend to eat a lot of starches, such as bread, pasta,
rice, and noodles. Y/N

I like to consume soft drinks, either with sugars or
artificially sweetened. Y/N

I tend to feel stuffed after eating a lot of my meals, whether
at home or in restaurants. Y/N

I like eating dessert, and I don't usually skip it. Y/N

Hormone Levels

I drink a lot of coffee, but I still wish I had more energy. Y/N

I often feel dizzy when I stand up. Y/N

I am a woman at least forty-five years of age, and I can tell
that my hormone levels fluctuate or are declining (or I am
now undergoing hormone-replacement therapy). Y/N

I am a woman at least forty-five years of age, and my energy
levels have noticeably decreased in recent years. Y/N

I am a woman at least forty-five years of age, and I've started
to gain weight that I just can't take off. Y/N

I am a man at least forty-five years of age, and my energy
levels and sexual desire have decreased in recent years. Y/N

I am a man, and I have fatty or enlarged breasts. Y/N

Illnesses and Medications

I have been diagnosed with or treated for a serious disease,
such as (but not limited to) heart disease, cancer, arthritis,
fibromyalgia, or chronic fatigue syndrome. Y/N

I have undergone surgery for a medical condition sometime
during the last five years.   Y/N

I have undergone open-heart surgery.   Y/N

I have undergone chemotherapy or radiation
treatment for cancer.   Y/N

I have prediabetes, type 2 diabetes, or hypoglycemia.   Y/N

I take one to two prescription drugs each day.   Y/N

I take three or more prescription drugs each day.   Y/N

I specifically take a statin drug (for example, Lipitor) for
cholesterol or an antidepressant (such as Prozac,
Zoloft, or Paxil).   Y/N

During the last three years, I have had to be a caregiver for
someone who had a serious disease or was dying.   Y/N

Aging

I've tended to gain more weight as I've gotten older.   Y/N

I get sleepy after meals, and I never used to.   Y/N

I feel that I'm more fatigued at my age than I should be.   Y/N

I think that my age might be a big factor in my fatigue.   Y/N

I was told by my doctor that some of my health problems are
related to my age.   Y/N

I could easily say that the older I get, the more tired I feel. Y/N

Interpretation: The more Y (yes) answers in each of the five circles points to the importance of those specific areas in causing your fatigue. For example, if you answered a lot of questions under "Eating Habits" with a Y but marked few Ys in the other categories, this would suggest that your diet is the main factor in your fatigue. It might help if you visualize the "Eating Habits" circle as being larger in your life than the other circles are. At this point, you may not understand how some of these questions relate to fatigue, but the links will become clear as you read on.

What You Should Expect

This questionnaire and the next five chapters will give you the information and the tools to regain the energy you need to pursue the life you want.

In chapter 1, I describe how stress decreases your energy and sets the stage for the other circles of fatigue, thus resulting in the Fatigue Syndrome. As incredible as it might sound, many people aren't even aware of how stressed they are and how it affects their lives and energy levels.

In chapter 2, I show that some so-called energy foods actually have the opposite effect and lead to low-energy "crashes." Nutrition is important because it forms the chemical basis of our biology and our energy production. Yet our eating habits are often influenced by stress. I recommend foods and eating habits that will naturally and gently boost and maintain your energy.

In chapter 3, I explain how changes in hormone levels—particularly, low levels of adrenal and thyroid hormones—can lower your energy. Age- and stress-related changes in hormones can powerfully affect your energy levels, and they can also have an impact on your weight and mental sharpness. Certain nutrients and eating habits can influence hormone levels. In this chapter, I will help you identify possible hormone imbalances and then encourage you to discuss specific tests and prescriptions with your physician.

In chapter 4, I focus on how serious illnesses, medications, and medical therapies can reduce energy levels and lead to the Fatigue Syndrome. Chronic illnesses are usually the long-term consequences of poor lifestyle habits, nutritional imbalances, and hormonal issues. Many serious illnesses, however, such as diabetes, chronic fatigue syndrome, fibromyalgia, cardiovascular disease, cancer, and infections, add to your total burden of fatigue. Furthermore, many medical treatments increase muscle weakness, mental fuzziness, and fatigue.

In chapter 5, I address the fifth circle of fatigue, that of aging. Aging puts additional pressures on the first four circles of fatigue. Even if you're in relatively good health, a fifty-year-old body has experienced more wear and tear than a twenty-year-old body has. When we were younger, we could tolerate a certain amount of intentional abuse to our bodies, such as staying up all night or getting drunk. With age, we become less tolerant of such abuses. Although the aging process entails specific biological changes that reduce our energy levels, we can minimize the effects of aging and enhance our built-in energy-production processes.

In part 2, I describe very specific eating habits, as well as menu plans, that will help maintain your energy levels. I'll discuss using nutritional supplements, suggest strategies to improve the quality of your sleep, and encourage you to adopt an easy program of physical activity. All of my suggestions should lead to a reduction in your fatigue and an improvement in energy.

Breakfast Boosts Stan's Energy Levels

Stan was a property manager, so he was frequently on the move. He usually had a very light breakfast, such as a bowl of soup or some toast. By 10 a.m., he'd be tired and hungry. And by lunchtime, Stan would be absolutely famished and would overeat, then feel like taking a nap.

I suggested that he start the day with a little protein, such as a poached egg or a couple of slices of turkey and cheese, along with a little fresh fruit. He did so, and on the very first day of eating a protein-centered breakfast, he called to tell me that he didn't feel tired by mid-morning—and that he wasn't overly hungry by noon. He had a light lunch, such as a chicken Caesar salad, and then kept working until the end of the day.

How quickly will you feel, and benefit from, this new surge of energy? Faster than you might imagine. In my nutrition coaching, I have consistently found that some of the simplest dietary changes lead to a newfound sense of energy and mental focus on the first day. If someone had told me years ago that I could improve my energy levels in only one day, I would not have believed it. Yet my clients have told me over and over again how happy they are to finally have the energy to do everything they want. You, too, can have optimal energy and defeat the Fatigue Syndrome.

Part One

Understanding the Fatigue Syndrome

The Five Circles of Fatigue

chapter 1

Stress and Fatigue

S tress is the single lifestyle factor that leads, both directly and indirectly, to a downward shift in your energy levels. It is in so many ways
the throttle that drives you into the other four circles of fatigue and deep
into the Fatigue Syndrome.

Dealing with the stress in your life is crucial to regaining the energy
you want. Whatever the other causes might be for your fatigue, you'll
have a much greater improvement in your energy level if you simultaneously tackle the stress that drags you down. I'll explain how stress affects
your energy and, later in the book, offer tips for controlling stress.

Many of us get so wrapped up in dealing with our day-to-day stresses—
most commonly related to work, deadlines, commuting, chores, and personal relationships—that we often don't even realize when we're totally
stressed out. That's the sinister nature of stress, because feeling pressured
encourages more reactive behavior than contemplation or proactive
thinking does. We end up running through our day-to-day activities like
a hamster spinning on its wheel, and we often go in circles, too. With all

of the things we have to do and all of the distractions that consume our attention and energy, stress becomes the norm, and it's difficult to even remember what normal once was.

Does this sound like your life? If it does, it may be a primary cause of your fatigue.

When you feel stressed, day in and day out, everything about your natural biology goes out of alignment. The effects of stress are like a shock wave that ripples through every part of the body, and stress hormones set in motion still other changes that will contribute to your feeling tired or wiped out. The first step is to recognize the things that stress you, and then you must learn to change them — or manage them better than you do.

What Exactly Is Stress?

We all hear the word *stress*, but what is it, really? I describe it as an unhealthy demand on your body or mind, something that pushes you beyond your normal equilibrium. Of course, some stresses are good for you, in that they can encourage creativity, problem solving, and productivity. But negative stresses push you in uncomfortable and unnatural ways and take a toll on your physical, mental, and emotional health — and, along the way, on your energy levels. They disrupt your equilibrium, your biological and biochemical balance, and whatever type of steadiness you strive for in your day-to-day life.

Most stresses seem to come from other people or from situations you are in, but many stresses actually originate in your own head or from your actions. People routinely internalize work and personal stresses, essentially bringing them from the outside to the inside. In fact, one could easily argue that nearly all stresses are internal because, unless your life is in immediate danger, it is your response to people and events that generates your stress. (You can, after all, simply ignore people's words or actions that contribute to your feelings of stress.) Some people are especially good at generating their own stress and anxiety when there should be none, such as by feeling compelled to e-mail or text when they should be sleeping or driving. Others seem to excel in creating a lot of chaos or commotion in their lives when none, again, needs to exist. Whatever the source of your stress, it can affect your moods (making you irritable or depressed) and your sleep habits, health, and energy levels. Quite simply, stress can and does wear you out.

Our Stress Response

The sudden onset of a negative stress triggers what biologists call the fight-or-flight response. This ancient part of our biology instantly prepares us to either fight for our survival or run for our lives, as if we were face-to-face with a tiger. A sudden and unexpected stress (these days, a sudden loud noise or someone yelling at us) triggers a near-instant secretion of adrenaline, a hormone that immediately increases our heart rate, quickens our reflexes, and sets other physiological changes in motion.

People, however, have come to differ from animals in their stress response. Scientist Robert Sapolsky, Ph.D., who wrote *Why Zebras Don't Get Ulcers*, has explained that when a tiger chases a deer, the deer's adrenaline levels surge and provide the muscles with extra energy to run. If the deer escapes, its adrenaline surge quickly dissipates, and the animal resumes grazing. It is rare for animals in the wild to experience chronic stress, the type that people now deal with almost every day for years and decades.

The truth is that you and I are not likely to ever come face-to-face with a tiger in the wild or to ever be victimized by a criminal. Instead, we live in a world filled with chronic work and home stresses of one sort or another. Under these circumstances, our bodies shift from making adrenaline to generating large amounts of cortisol, the principal long-term stress hormone. This is a primary factor in the Fatigue Syndrome.

Both adrenaline and cortisol are produced by two small adrenal glands, which sit atop our kidneys. When we're fighting stress, our cortisol levels stay elevated to help buffer the effects. When we exhaust our ability to make cortisol, however, we slip into adrenal exhaustion, sometimes called adrenal burnout. Coffee and other stimulants can

> ### *quick tip*
> ### The Connection between Stress, Inflammation, and the Fatigue Syndrome
>
> When we feel stressed, our bodies release a variety of pro-inflammatory cytokines, including interleukin-6 and C-reactive protein. Cytokines are highly specialized chemicals that can initiate and sustain an inflammatory response. They're important, biologically, because they tell cells to secrete still other infection-fighting chemicals. Yet the release of cytokines also causes fatigue. That's one way stress contributes to our feeling tired.

keep us going when our adrenals are exhausted, but at that point, we truly are stressed out and hobbling through life. I'll return to the subject of adrenal exhaustion in chapter 3.

Stress, Overweight, and Fatigue

Stress places a greater demand on your ability to make adrenal hormones. Stress also triggers a near-immediate shift in your eating habits, however, so it quickly affects both the first and the second circles of fatigue. Faced with a pressing deadline, you may delay eating or completely skip lunch or dinner. As your blood sugar drops, your liver will try to compensate by releasing some stored sugar, called glycogen. Within a couple of hours, though, you will likely experience a "blood sugar crash" (hypoglycemia) because you haven't eaten. The combination of low blood sugar and stress hormones can alter your brain chemistry, making you more irritable, impatient, and physically weak or shaky.

Many people sense what's happening and will try to boost their blood sugar levels by eating some type of junk food—a candy bar, an energy bar, or fast food (such as McDonald's). Yet these quick fixes are neither healthy nor a long-term solution. Foods that are high in sugars and processed starches rapidly boost blood sugar levels, but this sharp rise usually precipitates another blood sugar crash within an hour or two. I'll explain more about eating habits and fatigue in the next chapter.

Over a period of years, the combination of chronic stress, poor eating habits, and up-and-down blood sugar levels leads to persistent and chronic feelings of fatigue and a full-blown Fatigue Syndrome. Many people respond by drinking more coffee and other caffeine-containing stimulants. It is no coincidence that since the 1990s, as work pressures became more intense, so many people and businesses went from forty-hour weeks to 24/7—and Starbucks grew at a phenomenal rate. Coffee kept everyone going. As our nation's eating habits deteriorated in other ways, the number of people who were overweight or prediabetic (characterized by elevated glucose and insulin levels) grew to what are now considered epidemic levels. Fatigue and poor mental concentration are among the chief symptoms of prediabetes and type 2 diabetes.

Sharp blood sugar fluctuations make for frequent and powerful hunger pangs, which lead to overeating, worsening both prediabetes and feelings of fatigue. Furthermore, the levels of two hormones, cortisol and insulin, increase under stress. The combination of these hormones is especially effective for storing extra calories as belly fat, particularly when people eat a lot of sugars and starches. Sadly, three of every four Americans are now overweight or obese. In Great Britain, two of every three adults are overweight or obese, and similar trends are occurring in other nations as they acquire Western day-to-day stresses and eating habits.

In many ways, being overweight—especially around the tummy area—is a marker of stress, poor eating habits, and fatigue. Yet belly fat doesn't simply hang around someone's middle, looking ugly. It is what doctors call visceral fat, a particularly insidious type of fat that wraps around internal organs and is difficult to get rid of without a person's making major changes in eating habits and exercise. It is metabolically active tissue, meaning that it functions much like any other organ, except that it doesn't do anything good. It is also a visible sign of insulin resistance, a type of prediabetes.

Belly fat secretes a variety of inflammation-promoting substances, including interleukin-6 and C-reactive protein, which circulate throughout the body and increase the risk of heart disease, cancer, Alzheimer's, arthritis, allergies, asthma, and other diseases. This type of fat serves as a magnet for white blood cells, which intermingle with the fat cells and secrete still more pro-inflammatory molecules. Having belly fat also increases a person's odds of developing fatty liver, which interferes with normal liver function, blood sugar regulation, and the breakdown of harmful chemicals. It's a slippery slope, and being only ten pounds over-weight can begin a vicious cycle of overeating and fatigue, resulting in the Fatigue Syndrome.

Stress and the Other Circles of Fatigue

Nutrients provide the foundation of your biochemistry, and when you don't eat nutritious foods, all manner of biochemical processes become impaired. The consequences are rarely immediate, but they do become more obvious over a period of months or years. For example, a low intake of certain nutrients, particularly vitamin C and the B-vitamin pantothenic acid, impairs your ability to make adrenal hormones, which help insulate you against stress. Similarly, a low intake of protein, iodine, and selenium impairs your ability to make thyroid hormones.

When you are chronically stressed, your body makes more of your stimulating, or "upper," neurotransmitters, such as adrenaline, nor-adrenaline, and dopamine. Adrenaline and noradrenaline are made by your brain and by your adrenal glands, and they share many of the same nutritional building blocks needed by your thyroid hormones. When you wear out your ability to make these neurotransmitters and hormones, you lose much of your ability to buffer stress. Your body starts to buckle under the weight of that stress, and adrenal exhaustion and low thyroid activity are among the consequences that rob you of energy and leave you feeling fatigued. (I discuss these hormone issues in greater detail in chapter 3.)

Stress and poor eating habits (including food sensitivities) are well established as triggers in diseases such as irritable bowel syndrome and asthma, probably because they trigger the release of pro-inflammatory chemicals called cytokines. The combination of stress, poor nutrition, and altered hormone levels increases the risk of developing more serious diseases, such as chronic fatigue syndrome, heart disease, Alzheimer's, and cancer. Many of the drugs used to treat diseases can cause fatigue, which can range from mild to debilitating. Furthermore, serious diseases and medications can affect your appetite and therefore your nutritional intake, as well as your hormone levels. All of these factors are exacerbated with age, in large part because your body's biochemistry and physiology become less efficient with age.

Incredibly, stress makes us look older, too. Amy Wechsler, M.D., of New York City, is board certified in both psychiatry and dermatology, and she has pointed out that stress hormones affect the skin, which is another way that stress affects the aging process. According to Wechsler, adrenaline reduces blood circulation to the skin, which eventually affects the complexion and the skin tone. High levels of cortisol, the long-term stress hormone, interfere with the production of collagen (the body's chief protein) and elastin, both of which are crucial for maintaining healthy, flexible, wrinkle-free skin. Stress can literally age the skin by years.

There are plenty of reasons to deal with the stress in your life!

Two Common but Ignored Causes of Stress-Related Fatigue

There are many different sources of stress in our lives, but for now I would like to focus on two very common but often unrecognized stress inducers: multitasking and personal technologies. Both are usually considered ways to increase our productivity or ability to stay connected with others, but they can quickly get out of hand, distract us, interfere with sleep, and end up being a major drain on our energy levels.

How Multitasking Contributes to Fatigue

Several years ago, I was a guest on a couple of live radio shows sponsored by Martha Stewart's *Body & Soul* magazine. As the host and I fielded calls from listeners, it became clear that the callers were leading very much the same life: they were moms calling from cell phones, with small children in the car, trying to juggle the demands of work, errands, the chaos in the backseat, and thinking about what to make for dinner. They were overwhelmed by what they had to do, and they were totally stressed out. I thought of the 1983 film *Koyaanisqatsi*, directed by Godfrey Reggio and musically scored by Philip Glass. *Koyaanisqatsi* (pronounced koy-ahn-is-kat-see) is a Hopi word meaning "life out of balance."

The radio show wasn't an isolated example. If you pay attention to how people walk, drive, stand in line at supermarkets, and even step into elevators, it becomes clear that nearly everyone is time stressed. There aren't enough hours in the day to do everything they must. People walk and drive fast, run red lights, eat while driving, are often impatient and rude while standing in line, and step into elevators before letting people exit. It seems to get worse, year after year, with cell phone calls, texting, and e-mailing while driving.

My father, in his simple way, would have described such frenetic activity as being like "a chicken running around with its head cut off." This is what chronic stress does to us, unless we make efforts to be mindful of its effect and modulate its impact. When we're stressed, our brains are simply reacting, not weighing the forces bearing down on us. We're like the deer running for its life.

People multitask—that is, do two or more activities at once—to keep up with everything they have to do. We've all been told, or have somehow come to believe, that multitasking increases our productivity. It certainly seems to be true—we'll get more done if we do two things at the same time.

It's not true, though. Multitasking is a myth that so many businesses hold to as if it were a religious doctrine. Just because people do things in a more frenetic way does not mean they're accomplishing more. Study after study has shown that multitasking actually reduces productivity and increases the risk of people making mistakes. The reason is that the brain takes anywhere from a few seconds to fifteen minutes to acclimate after switching gears. All that multitasking really does is foster a type of hyperactive behavior in adults that we discourage and medicate in children. It is mentally fatiguing to multitask. It is also far more efficient, as quaint and old-fashioned as it might seem, to do one task at a time and to devote ourselves to finishing it before moving to another.

You might think that frequent multitaskers are better able to juggle more than one task, compared with the average person. Yet that's not the case, either. A 2009 study published in the *Proceedings of the National Academy of Sciences* reported that people who multitasked a lot (compared with those who did so only a little) were actually more likely to be distracted and less able to ignore meaningless information. Less than 3 percent of people are efficient multitaskers, which means that the vast majority of folks are not very good at it; they just think they are.

Still other studies have shown that multitasking prompts the same stressful increases in adrenaline and cortisol as a fight-or-flight response. So instead of easing your time stress, multitasking makes it worse. And the more stressed and anxious you are, the more likely you will feel fatigued, and the greater your risk of developing adrenal exhaustion and other health problems.

You may be very skeptical of what I write here, but if you still have doubts, consider a simple illustration: think about all of the times you have been behind a slow driver who was talking on his cell phone. The phone conversation typically gets far more attention than the driving does, so the driver just putters along well under the speed limit, and you end up speeding around him and swearing under your breath. Whether you want to admit it or not, you're no different when driving and talking on your phone, and hands-free devices don't seem to improve the situation. Multitasking merely creates more frenzied behavior, adds to your feelings of stress, and eventually contributes to your feeling fatigued.

How Personal Technologies Can Cause Stress and Fatigue

One major source of multitasking stress in recent years has been bred by technology addiction—literally, an addiction to e-mailing and texting, tweeting, and surfing the Net. The addictive nature of personal technologies chips away at our energy levels, reduces regenerative quiet times, and interferes with restful sleep. Interestingly enough, technology addiction had its roots in the 1970s with early computer and video games, such as Pac Man and Space Invaders. Now there are hundreds of games for computers, Playstations, Xboxes, and smart phones. Even e-mail, Facebook, texting, and tweeting can be the equivalent of interactive and addictive computer games that demand an immediate response from us.

People commonly remain oblivious to how they interact with personal technologies, and it's not just the loudmouth who unwittingly shares his cell phone conversation with everyone else in the supermarket line or slows the line by yakking away when he should be swiping a credit card. I often find myself stepping around people who are walking down the street and e-mailing or texting on their BlackBerries and iPhones. They stumble around like zombies from a horror film, a point astutely made in the first few minutes of the movie *Shaun of the Dead*. The sad truth is that just as people cannot devote equal parts of their minds to driving and talking on the phone, a lot of people simply can't walk and use their smart phones at the same time. This might strike you as funny, but such an obsession with personal technologies actually adds to your stress burden.

For many people, it is near impossible not to immediately respond to a cell phone call, a text, or an e-mail. Ignoring a call or a text triggers feelings of stress and anxiety—a characteristic of obsessive-compulsive disorder. Conflicts inevitably arise between those with technology addictions and other people. In many homes, parents and children are busy e-mailing and texting while having dinner at the same table (instead of maybe talking with one another). The glow of cell phones and text messaging has become such a distraction that in some theaters, ushers will evict people for using their phones during a movie. Across the country, a number of bicyclists have been struck or killed by car drivers who believed they could text while driving.

On one trip to New York City, I found myself standing next to a man while waiting to cross the intersection. Rather, *I* was waiting to cross the intersection. With earbuds in his ears, he was listening to music, typing feverishly on his phone's keyboard, and trying to cross against the red light as yellow taxis whizzed by within inches of him. He'd step forward into traffic, then back, then forward again. I kept hoping that he didn't get hit by a car right in front of me. (Luckily, he didn't!) There is no other way to describe such behavior other than as a form of obsessive-compulsive disorder or addiction.

Why are personal technologies so addictive, and why do so many people now crave electronic (as opposed to direct human) stimulation? Two lengthy articles published in the *New York Times* in June 2010 explored some of the reasons. First, personal technologies trigger an ancient biological impulse to respond immediately to a situation, as impulsive as that response might be in today's world. Second, the excitement of the response to an e-mail or a text message is related to the release of dopamine, the neurotransmitter that creates a powerful but brief "high" feeling. Dopamine is extraordinarily addictive and is the chemical behind sexual and shopper's highs, as well as cocaine's and methamphetamine's action on the brain. It's easy to feed a dopamine addiction by responding immediately to e-mails or texts, and the lack of this chemical stimulus leads to feelings of boredom.

The *New York Times'* articles addressed another aspect of personal technology addiction. Spouses (or domestic partners) can be frequently distracted by interactive technologies, and these distractions are capable of damaging interpersonal relationships. Picture two people in bed with their laptops, when they might actually be having more fun sexually. But the real casualty may be children, who get the short shrift in a competition with their parents' personal technologies. When parents are busy with their computers, iPads, and smart phones, their children often feel abandoned, hurt, and jealous. The irony, of course, is that many parents are concerned about their children's addiction to personal technologies but remain oblivious about their own technology addiction and its effect on child development.

Whether you have small children or not, between computers and cell phones, it is now so effortless to e-mail or text late at night—a habit that so obviously interferes with sleep. This is the grip that technology has on us, unless we exercise great care and remember that we always have a choice between answering and not answering, reading and not reading, responding and not responding when we hear a ring or a ping. We also have the option, lest we forget, of simply turning a phone off.

In the next chapter, I focus on how stress affects our eating habits and how the specific foods we eat can either contribute to the Fatigue Syndrome or help us maintain steady and strong energy levels.

chapter 2

Eating Habits and Fatigue

The foods and the specific nutrients we consume form the biochemical foundation of our bodies and enable us to make energy. Some nutrients serve as fuel, while others function as essential parts of our biological engines. Similarly, certain foods and nutrients enhance our ability to make energy, while others have the opposite effect and interfere with our bodies' energy production, thus contributing to the Fatigue Syndrome. For these reasons, our eating habits form the second circle of fatigue.

Odds are that you know at least some of the differences between healthy and unhealthy eating habits, although you might not always follow good dietary practices on a daily basis. Any discussion of food, however, is ultimately about more than simple nutrition. Eating habits do not exist in a vacuum, and the foods we choose to eat are shaped by our upbringing and education and strongly influenced by advertising, peer pressure, and the time that we have available for eating. Stress is a major factor because, when we feel pressured or anxious, our eating habits quickly slide, however noble our intentions. When we skip meals and later succumb to sweets and fast foods, our physical and mental energy rises and falls during the course of a day, instead of holding steady.

Unfortunately, much of what we have heard since childhood about "energy foods" and "energy drinks" has been wrong, and we end up following bad nutritional advice in our efforts to boost our energy. For example, nearly all of us were at one time taught that sugar is an energy food. Although the idea is technically true in a narrow biochemical sense, it grossly distorts the role that dietary sugars and starches (non-sugar carbohydrates) play in the body's production of energy. There are many reasons for this misinformation, not the least of which is the desire of many companies to earn billions of dollars annually from distorting the facts and in their marketing of unhealthy foods.

The late Hugh D. Riordan, M.D., a friend and a pioneer in nutritional medicine, astutely observed that many people overeat in an attempt to increase their energy. When they feel tired or sleepy, they think they can get a quick boost from eating a sugary or carb-rich food. Yet these foods actually create a rebound that leads to repeated and greater feelings of tiredness and sets the stage for food addictions, overeating, and overweight.

The confusion about energy foods and drinks has had far-reaching consequences beyond that of people simply feeling tired much of the time. The Fatigue Syndrome can be a harbinger of serious diseases, including diabetes, heart disease, cancer, and Alzheimer's disease—all of which are known to be related to dietary habits. Furthermore, fatigue often robs us of the motivation to take important steps to improve our health. Many people simply don't have the energy to cook fresh foods (instead of microwaving packaged foods), although fresh foods will usually contribute to higher energy levels. Ominously, as American-style fast food and convenience foods—which are anything but fresh—have been marketed around the world, they have created a vicious cycle of overeating and fatigue. Meanwhile, the healthiest energy-generating foods are almost always overlooked.

How Our Bodies Make Energy

To understand the biology of energy and fatigue, it helps if we grasp the basics of how the body generates energy from the fundamental building blocks of food, as well as why energy is so important to our overall health.

In the 1930s, Nobel laureate Albert V. Szent-Györgyi, M.D., Ph.D., captured the essence of the explanation by writing that energy was the "currency" of life. Szent-Györgyi was referring specifically to energy produced in individual cells. Your body contains approximately 70 trillion cells, and their collective energy output is literally what keeps you alive and moving. Without energy, life cannot exist.

So, how did energy become so integrated into life? Biologists believe that millions of years ago, two types of early cells merged into one to create an interdependent cell within a cell. The energy powerhouse was the mitochondrion, and today every cell of our bodies contains mitochondria. Mitochondria break down some of the basic constituents of our food, such as glucose and fat, to make energy. In fact, mitochondria even contain their own genes, separate from the rest of our genes. I'll describe the nutritional requirements of mitochondria and energy later in the book, but for now, I just want to explain a little about how they influence your energy levels.

A cell contains anywhere from one to thousands of mitochondria, depending on the energy requirements of that type of cell. Muscle cells, heart cells (a specific type of muscle cell), liver cells, and brain cells are among the most metabolically active cells in the body, and they also contain the largest number of mitochondria. These cells need this many mitochondria because they have higher energy requirements than, say, skin or lung cells. The average person's heart beats around three trillion times in a lifetime, an enormous sustained effort over seventy-five or so years. If you exercise consistently, you can increase both the number and the size of your muscle cells, and your muscle cells will respond to the demands of exercising by producing more mitochondria. If you do not exercise, your muscle cells will contain comparatively fewer mitochondria.

In the early 1960s, doctors discovered that some people are born with mitochondrial myopathies—muscle diseases caused by damaged mitochondrial DNA. Depending on the specific type of DNA damage, mitochondrial myopathies can affect energy production in the heart, the brain, and the skeletal muscles (that is, muscles of the arms, the back, and the legs). Severe mental retardation results from some types of mitochondrial damage, while overwhelming fatigue and droopy eyelids (which are usually evident in infancy or childhood) result from still other forms of mitochondrial DNA damage. In some cases the mitochondrial myopathies were inherited, and in others they were congenital.

By 1988, researchers realized that *acquired* mitochondrial damage accelerates the aging process and boosts the risk of developing various serious diseases, such as cancer, neurodegenerative diseases, and certain types of heart disease. This link between mitochondria and aging should not be entirely surprising because both muscle mass and energy levels decline as people get older, just as the functioning of high-energy organs (for example, the heart and the brain) also deteriorates with age. Age-related damage to mitochondria interferes with our ability to use food molecules for energy, and, as we become less active, we lose both muscle cells and the number of mitochondria within the remaining muscle cells. Many researchers now believe that diminishing mitochondrial function is primarily responsible for the aging process and the failure of specific organs, such as the heart, the brain, and the immune system.

A small number of physicians have focused on reversing mitochondrial myopathies, as well as cardiomyopathy and heart failure (diseases that involve a lack of energy in heart cells), with specific vitamin-like nutrients, such as coenzyme Q10 (CoQ10) and L-carnitine, to enhance mitochondrial function. Similarly, Parkinson's disease and other neurological conditions appear to be related, at least in part, to a catastrophic loss of energy in brain cells. Perhaps not surprisingly, then, studies have found that large amounts of supplemental CoQ10 can slow the progression of Parkinson's disease by enhancing energy production in the brain.

It's important to recognize that CoQ10 and L-carnitine are not burned for energy. Instead, they play roles in the biochemical machinery that does burn glucose and fat for energy. L-carnitine helps transport fats into mitochondria, where they are, in a manner of speaking, combusted for energy, much in the way that a fuel injector delivers gasoline into an automobile engine. Electrons, a type of subatomic particle, carry much of the energy within mitochondria, and CoQ10 helps move those electrons within mitochondria. I'll discuss these and other mitochondrial nutrients in greater detail in chapter 6.

Sugar Is an Anti-Energy, Fat-Producing Food

Returning to the discussion of dietary sugars, most people believe that sugar (a generic term for sucrose and high-fructose corn syrup) is our best energy food. That's part of the reason why many people reach for something sweet, such as a candy bar or an energy bar, when they need a lift. Yet sugar, again, is really an anti-energy food.

When the body does not burn sugar and sugarlike carbs (think in terms of breads, pastas, pizza crusts, and bagels), these foodstuffs are converted to fat and stored in the belly, the buttocks, the liver, and the muscles, or they remain in the blood as cholesterol and triglycerides. This situation reflects a common problem in our sedentary society, in which people spend large amounts of time in cars or trucks, at a desk, or in front of a computer or a television screen. The lack of physical activity decreases the number of sugar- and fat-burning mitochondria in cells, which further contributes to a reduction in energy-producing capacity. The situation is compounded by the consumption of large amounts of foods that contain sugars, sugarlike carbs, and junk fats (for example, trans fats, corn oil, and soybean oil). All of these foods are low in the specific nutrients (such as B vitamins, CoQ10, and L-carnitine) that your body needs to burn them for energy. As a consequence, sugars and carbs are even more likely to be stored as cholesterol or body fat.

At best, sugar- and carb-rich foods are nothing more than empty calories. With three of every four adults and one of every three children now overweight or obese, few people can afford to consume nutritionally void calories, at least if they want to maintain some semblance of

---

quick tip
What about Sugar Substitutes?

Aspartame is the most common sugar substitute that is used in diet soft drinks or added to coffee. It is chemically similar to phenylalanine, the amino acid building block of the neurotransmitter phenylethylamine. Aspartame is a stimulant, and, like other stimulants, it can eventually contribute to feelings of fatigue. In addition, it can cause anxiety, migraine headaches, and mood alterations. Aspartame and other sugar substitutes might actually increase our desire for sweet foods, which can be a factor in fatigue.

---

health. Our modern-day epidemic of overweight and obesity points in part to a gross imbalance in energy metabolism. An analogy might be pouring fuel into an engine that doesn't work.

Is Your Fatigue Related to Prediabetes?

One of the most common causes of persistent feelings of physical and mental fatigue is undiagnosed prediabetes or poorly controlled type 2 diabetes. The root of these conditions is primarily dietary—again, too many sugars and sugarlike carbs—and, in most cases, these forms of diabetes can be partially or completely reversed with improved eating habits. It's important for you to understand how blood sugar affects fatigue and energy before I suggest specific dietary improvements.

As I explained in my previous book, *Stop Prediabetes Now*, sugars and sugarlike carbs are absorbed very quickly, leading to either a steep rise in blood sugar levels or extreme fluctuations between high and low blood sugar levels. How do blood sugar problems contribute to your feeling tired? When blood sugar rises rapidly, such as after you consume a candy bar, an ice cream cone, or a carb-rich meal, your body responds by secreting insulin, a hormone that transports glucose out of the bloodstream and into cells, where the glucose is either stored as fat or burned for energy. In many people, blood sugar and insulin levels oscillate every couple of hours, so that people have alternating periods of low and high energy (rather than steady energy) levels during the day.

The low-energy effect is most noticeable after lunch or dinner, when many people become mentally fuzzy and feel like taking a nap. Several years ago, researchers discovered that high blood sugar levels turn off the brain's production of orexins, a family of chemicals that normally helps keep us alert. Many people incorrectly attribute their tiredness after a meal to low blood sugar (hypoglycemia), and they often respond by eating something sweet, which causes blood sugar levels to spike higher and exacerbate the fatigue.

After a number of years—the time line varies from person to person—the body's cells stop responding to insulin, and both blood sugar and insulin levels remain elevated. At this point, people are insulin resistant and are well on the way to developing type 2 diabetes. At the same time, extreme elevations of blood sugar and insulin prompt the secretion of several inflammation-promoting chemicals called cytokines, particularly interleukin-6 and C-reactive protein, which initiate an "inflammatory cascade" that also contributes to people's feeling tired.

Sugar-related fatigue is one reason why many people have difficulty waking up in the morning. This is especially true of those who routinely eat late-night meals or snack after dinner, such as when they're watching television. Their blood sugar remains elevated overnight, so they feel tired when the alarm clock rings. In addition, they are not hungry in the morning (again, because their blood sugar is elevated), so they skip breakfast. Skipping breakfast further interferes with normal blood sugar levels and sets the stage for their overeating later in the day and feeling tired. Recent research has also shown that eating at the "wrong" times, such as late at night, alters the circadian rhythm and the activity of circadian-dependent genes, all of which can disturb sleep habits, lead to weight gain, and reduce energy levels.

It's not only the steady consumption of bread, pasta, candy bars, and various sweets. Soft drinks also contribute to the blood sugar overload—a typical 12-ounce can contains approximately 12 teaspoons of sugars, and a 64-ounce bottle has around one-half cup of sugars. The

---

quick tip
Overweight, Obesity, and Diabetes

An estimated 100 million Americans have some form of prediabetes. Diabetes and overweight are tightly intertwined, and obesity increases the likelihood of developing type 2 diabetes by eighty times. Three of every four American adults are overweight or obese. Each year 1 million Americans graduate from having prediabetes to full-blown type 2 diabetes.

---

amount of sugar is roughly equivalent to a physician-administered glucose-tolerance test, so one could wryly argue that soft drink companies make a business of dispensing medical tests without a license. Various fruit juices and yogurt-based beverages can be just as bad as soft drinks, if not worse. Some contain large amounts of so-called natural sugars (for example, glucose and fructose), and others have large amounts of added high-fructose corn syrup.

Frequent and sharp blood sugar swings encourage junk food binges and food addictions. One clue to diagnosing prediabetes and type 2 diabetes is when someone has regular cravings for sugary or carb-rich foods or a penchant for eating sweet foods once or more daily. As blood sugar problems become more serious, the tongue's sensitivity to sweetness tends to decrease, so people will seek out more intense sources of sweetness to get their "sugar hit." Instead of adding one teaspoon of sugar to coffee, they might add two or three teaspoons. Or instead of eating one piece of chocolate, they might have three or four.

Coffee Is an Anti-Energy Drink

To combat morning fatigue and low-energy periods during the day, millions of people drink coffee or other caffeine-containing beverages, such as soft drinks and energy drinks. In small amounts, caffeine can have remarkable physical and neurological benefits. It quickly stimulates the secretion of adrenaline, an "upper" neurotransmitter that sharpens thinking. Caffeine also improves mood, concentration, energy, and reaction times. Studies have found that modest coffee consumption might even reduce the risk of diabetes and Parkinson's disease.

The association between coffee and the risk of heart disease and cancer, unfortunately, is murkier. Roughly half of Americans have an efficient version of the CYP1A2 liver enzyme, which breaks down 95 percent of the caffeine that enters the body. If you inherited the ability to make large amounts of CYP1A2 enzyme and consume modest amounts of coffee, you will actually have a lower than average risk of developing heart disease. If, however, you inherited an inefficient version of the CYP1A2 enzyme, coffee will increase your risk of heart disease.

If modest coffee consumption has a relatively neutral health effect, consuming large amounts can contribute to a host of health problems, regardless of whether you have an efficient or inefficient CYP1A2 enzyme. Large amounts of caffeine can lead to rebound fatigue, anxiety, erratic or rapid heartbeats, and overstimulation of the central nervous system, resulting in poor sleep.

Coffee has often been described as the most widely used—and abused—drug in the world. As our lives have become more stressful, we have become more dependent on coffee as a way of pushing our bodies and minds to accomplish all of the things we want to do. Nine out of every ten Americans now consume at least one or two cups of coffee daily, and four of those nine people consume four or more cups daily. This dependence on coffee frequently turns into a powerful addiction. Consider this online confession: "I am a Starbucks junkie. I need a good cup of java to keep me alive. I cannot live without it. Don't blame the coffee, it's just me."

If you consume coffee or other caffeinated beverages on a daily basis, and you feel fatigued, I know that you can't imagine giving up your coffee or energy drinks. But consuming excessive amounts of caffeine is like any other addiction. You may be lucky enough to draw the line at one or two cups daily, but odds are that you will eventually need the energy surge provided by larger amounts of caffeine.

So, what's a reasonable amount, and what's too much coffee or caffeine? The answer is very subjective. In my opinion, a cup or two of relatively weak coffee (providing 95 mg or less of caffeine per cup) in the morning is fine for many people—assuming that they also consume a protein-rich breakfast. Eating that breakfast is a very important caveat. Consuming adequate protein with breakfast (for example, an egg, a small amount of chicken or turkey, or a bowl of steel-cut oatmeal) helps temper the effect of caffeine on blood sugar and adrenaline.

Conversely, if you have coffee but skip breakfast or simply eat something sweet, you are literally using caffeine and sugar as drugs. Worse yet is ordering a grande (16-ounce) size of Starbucks brewed coffee, which provides a whopping 330 mg of caffeine. (A Starbucks 20-ounce venti size of coffee contains 500 mg of caffeine!) Furthermore, all types of coffee and other caffeine-containing beverages become much more problematic when consumed in the late afternoon or the evening, because they are more likely to keep you wired when you want to sleep. Even so-called decaffeinated coffee retains about 5 percent of its caffeine.

Can You Wean Yourself from Coffee?

People frequently ask me how to reduce their dependence on coffee. That's another sign of the addictive power of this beverage. The coffee habit is difficult but not impossible to break. The timing and the situation are crucial to success, as is taking a deep breath to deal with the fear of changing one of your habits.

I often suggest that heavy coffee drinkers work on giving up their drug at the beginning of a one- to two-week vacation. Being on a vacation removes people from the stress triggers that prompt caffeine consumption. Vacations also enable them to sleep late and nurse a possible withdrawal headache. If you develop a headache from giving up coffee, treat it with ibuprofen or aspirin but avoid caffeine-containing analgesics such as Excedrin. You might also be able to nap through the headache. During this time, do not consume black and green tea, soft drinks, or chocolate, which also contain caffeine.

Another option is to dilute your coffee and reduce the amount of caffeine you consume. You can do this by using half the amount of ground coffee when brewing it. Still another option is mixing your coffee with an equal amount of chicory root or Teecchino, both of which are tasty coffee substitutes sold at many natural food stores. For example, once you acclimate to a 50–50 blend of coffee and Teecchino, then you can reduce the amount of coffee a little more, so that the ratio is 40–60. Keep reducing the amount of coffee over two to four weeks until you can drink a cup of 100 percent pure Teecchino without experiencing any caffeine-withdrawal symptoms.

Yet another option is to buy a high-quality green tea, which will contain some caffeine, but its negative effects will likely be countered by L-theanine, a substance that is also found in the tea. L-theanine is a natural compound that has neurotransmitter-like effects, specifically improving both mental focus and promoting a sense of relaxation. L-theanine provides the flavor of green tea, and, unfortunately, most cheaper green tea brands contain little L-theanine. One of the highest-quality green teas is the awkwardly named "Catechin-Rich Green Tea," distributed by Miroku. (Catechins are a family of antioxidants found in green tea.) Each teabag yields a full pitcher of rich-flavored green tea, which can be served hot or iced. (See miroku-usa.com.) I brew a daily pitcher on my countertop and drink it throughout the day, and it does not affect my sleep.

---

quick tip
What Is Teecchino?

Teecchino is a coffee alternative that's completely caffeine-free. Although the ingredients vary somewhat among the ten flavors, all of them contain carob, barley, and chicory. Among the available flavors are java, mocha, hazelnut, vanilla nut, and almond amaretto. The products have been tested, and brewed cups do not contain any detectable amounts (less than 10 parts per million) of gluten. For more information, visit teecchino.com.

Energy Drinks and Caffeine Abuse

Caffeine has long been a key ingredient in the vast majority of soft drinks. Most traditional soft drinks, such as Coca-Cola and Pepsi, have 35 to 55 mg of caffeine in a 12-ounce serving, regardless of whether they are diet or regular drinks. Even some noncola soft drinks, such as Mountain Dew, contain comparable amounts of caffeine. Others, including 7-Up and Sprite, do not have any caffeine, although they may contain substantial amounts of sugars.

As dietary habits deteriorated, drinking a Coke or a Pepsi for breakfast became much more common, beginning in the 1980s. At that time and in the early 1990s, beverage companies began to market energy drinks more aggressively, and these beverages became popular among teenagers and twenty-somethings. Red Bull, which contains 76 mg of caffeine in a 12-ounce serving, was introduced in 1997 and has since become the top-selling energy drink. Red Bull and other energy drinks are more popular among men in their twenties and thirties, whereas middle-age and older folks still prefer coffee.

Some soft drinks and energy drinks contain herbs or vitamins, and a few experts have questioned their inclusion. That issue is really a subterfuge because the amounts of herbs or vitamins are usually small and nothing more than window dressing. The more serious issue is that energy drinks often provide significant amounts of both caffeine and sugars, inevitably leading to a low-energy rebound. For all of Red Bull's popularity, its caffeine content is pretty tame compared with many other popular energy drinks, such as Monster Energy (160 mg of caffeine in 16 ounces), SoBe No Fear (174 mg of caffeine in 16 ounces), Rockstar (240 mg of caffeine in 16 ounces), or Jolt (280 mg of caffeine in 23.5 ounces).

The company that makes 5-Hour Energy shots does not disclose the amount of caffeine in each 2-ounce shot, other than to state that it is the same amount found in "the leading premium coffee," presumably Starbucks. Granted, most of these energy drinks fall short of the amount of caffeine in an unsweetened grande-size Starbucks coffee (330 mg caffeine), but, again, the consumption of both caffeine and sugar is essentially a form of self-medication with two different drugs. Consider that a Starbucks venti-size (20-ounce) Peppermint Mocha Twist Frappuccino with whipped cream contains 55 mg of caffeine and 660 calories, including almost a quarter-pound of sugars. Some of Starbucks drinks have a little less sugar but more than twice the caffeine!

Worse is the cumulative effect of consuming multiple energy drinks, several cups of coffee, and various sweets, from candy bars to energy bars. The effects of large amounts of caffeine on the body can mimic anxiety attacks. And although small amounts of caffeine function as a stimulant, greater amounts of caffeine (especially when combined with sugars) can actually provoke the opposite effect—that of a downer.

In one study, British researchers found that after consuming a popular energy drink (30 mg of caffeine and 42 grams of sugars), people had slower reaction times and felt sleepy! Many studies have shown that large amounts of caffeine disrupt sleep and lead to sleepiness the next day, which creates a need for more caffeine. Still other research suggests that caffeine decreases the body's levels of several amino acids (protein constituents), a change that may alter mood and result in profound fatigue.

In the long term, consuming large amounts of caffeine (and trying to cope with various stresses and a lack of restful sleep) can contribute to adrenal exhaustion and full-blown Fatigue Syndrome. This is often the case with people who consume five or more cups of coffee, or several energy drinks, daily but still feel perpetually tired. (I'll discuss adrenal exhaustion in greater detail in the next chapter.) The bottom line is that there is a point of diminishing returns with excess caffeine. Yet as with other types of addiction, people often feel trapped by their dependence on caffeine and are afraid of the consequences of reducing their intake.

Soft Drink Consumption Leads to Muscle Fatigue and Weakness

Consuming soft drinks throughout the day can result in fatigue for reasons unrelated to sugar or caffeine rebound. Large amounts of glucose, fructose, or caffeine deplete the body's potassium, which results in muscle weakness, fatigue, and, in some cases, paralysis. Potassium is an essential dietary mineral that functions as an electrolyte, a compound needed for normal muscle function.

Low potassium and the consequent fatigue become most noticeable in people who consume several quarts (or liters) of soft drinks daily, particularly colas. Drinking large amounts of sugars and caffeine increases urination, alters potassium activity in cells, and produces still greater potassium losses from mild-to-severe diarrhea. It is very likely that the regular consumption of smaller amounts of colas also affects potassium activity.

In case histories described in the *International Journal of Clinical Practice*, doctors reported that muscle weakness and fatigue were reversed after the patients stopped consuming soft drinks. Sometimes these patients recovered quickly after also taking potassium supplements.

Giving Up Soft Drinks Boosts Jeannette's Energy Levels

Jeannette, age twenty-five, was about halfway through her first pregnancy. She went to her doctor complaining about severe fatigue, muscle weakness, loss of appetite, and soft stools. Laboratory tests indicated that she was low in potassium, a mineral involved in normal heart and muscle function.

Jeannette's doctor felt that her fatigue and other symptoms were related to low potassium levels. He asked about her eating habits, and she acknowledged having intense cravings for sugary foods and also said she was consuming three to four quarts of cola daily.

The doctor recommended that Jeannette stop having soft drinks and that she make other improvements in her diet. He also prescribed potassium supplements for a couple of weeks. Jeannette's energy bounced back within days of her making these changes.

Allergies, Foods, and Fatigue

Allergies to pollens are a common cause of fatigue; so are many of the prescription and nonprescription drugs, such as antihistamines and certain so-called nondrowsy medications, that people take to lessen allergy symptoms. Pollen allergies can interact with food sensitivities and increase feelings of fatigue.

Pollen allergies reflect an inappropriate immune system response to an innocuous substance. What causes this misguided immune response? Many scientists believe it is due to "molecular mimicry," meaning that the chemical structure of a pollen may bear similarities to a more threatening bacteria or virus. This theory, of course, does not answer the question of why some but not all people are allergic to ragweed, juniper, or other pollens. In certain people, this abnormal programming of the immune system (to react to pollens) is permanent, and in others, it can be moderated.

Whatever the cause, millions of people suffer from pollen allergies, which are commonly aggravated by food allergies (or food sensitivities) that people are unaware of. (For a more detailed discussion of allergies, please refer to my book *The Inflammation Syndrome*.) Food allergies can be very difficult to confirm with traditional medical tests, so a symptomatic response is often the most reliable guide. Complicating the diagnosis is that people are often addicted to the very foods they are allergic to. In other words, food cravings (such as for chocolate, bread, or pasta) suggest a food allergy. One clue to food allergies is to consider which foods you can't imagine living without. The answer will almost always points to the culprit food.

Food allergies have been called "the great mimicker" (as syphilis once was) because their symptoms can be so individualized and can resemble or exacerbate the symptoms of almost any health problem, including heart palpitations, arthritis, and depression. Sometimes people will experience a "crash" (that is, fall asleep) shortly after indulging in a problematic food, or they will wake up the next morning with an allergy "hangover." A food-allergy hangover can be eerily similar to an alcohol hangover, in which people feel being completely wiped out and headachy and have puffy dark circles under their eyes. This type of reaction certainly does not enhance their energy levels.

As if food allergies weren't complicated enough, some foods interact with pollens and worsen the allergic response and contribute to fatigue.

It should be no surprise that grains, which are related to grasses, can increase the discomfort of grass pollen allergies. These concomitant food/pollen allergies are a little like binary weapons; individually, they may provoke a mild reaction or none at all, whereas their combination triggers a strong response. If you have pollen allergies, you can probably lessen their intensity by avoiding their concomitant foods during allergy season.

For example,

- If you are sensitive to ragweed, avoid egg, dairy, and mint.
- If you are sensitive to grasses, avoid all legumes and grains.
- If you are sensitive to juniper and cedar, avoid beef and brewer's yeast.
- If you are sensitive to elm, avoid eggs and apples.
- If you are sensitive to dust, avoid oysters, clams, scallops, and possibly nuts.

If you have allergies and can reduce the symptoms they cause without resorting to antihistamines and other medications that contribute to sleepiness, you will be less likely to suffer from allergy-related fatigue. I favor two remedies. One is quercetin, an antioxidant found in apples and onions that may be helpful in dosages ranging from 1,000 mg to 2,000 mg daily. Quercetin is sold at most health food stores and also online. Another remedy is chromolyn sodium, which is a synthetic antioxidant similar to quercetin. Chromolyn sodium is a nasal spray that prevents cells in the nasal passages from releasing histamine, the substance that causes much of the discomfort with allergies. You can buy chromolyn sodium at most pharmacies.

Nutritional Deficiencies and Fatigue

A great many vitamins and minerals play important roles in the body's breakdown of food for energy, and low intake of these nutrients can also cause fatigue. Most likely, a deficiency of *any* nutrient will contribute to fatigue because it will interfere with a variety of normal biochemical processes. Yet several specific nutrient deficiencies stand out in terms of their relationship to the Fatigue Syndrome.

Vitamin C

In human studies conducted at the National Institutes of Health, in Bethesda, Maryland, Mark Levine, M.D., found that the first two symptoms of vitamin C deficiency were fatigue and irritability, two very common symptoms. Vitamin C is involved in the production of both physical and mental energy. It is needed to make L-carnitine (and related carnitine compounds), which is necessary to transport fats into mitochondria. Researchers at Arizona State University, Tempe, found that low vitamin C levels reduce the body's ability to burn calories during exercise and increase postexercise fatigue. Taking vitamin C supplements can restore the normal fat-burning abilities of mitochondria.

The vitamin is also needed to make our "upper" neurotransmitters, such as dopamine, norepinephrine, and epinephrine. A lack of vitamin C results in mental lethargy, which is likely due in part to low levels of these brain chemicals. In a recent study, Korean physicians gave 6 grams of vitamin C daily for two weeks to forty-four workers. By the end of the study, their levels of fatigue lessened by almost one-third. In addition, the workers' blood sugar and cortisol levels decreased, as did their liver enzymes (a sign of improved liver function).

Vitamin D

This vitamin is necessary for the body's production of muscle tissue and to regulate insulin and blood sugar levels. Most of the body's mitochondria are found in the muscles, and inadequate numbers of mitochondria impact energy levels. In fact, the symptoms of vitamin D deficiency are sometimes difficult to distinguish from those of chronic fatigue syndrome, which include muscle weakness, fatigue, and depression.

A few years ago, doctors generally believed that falls and fractures in the elderly were due to weak bones. Current thinking is that falls might be the result of weak muscles, which become unable to support the weight of the body. Both physical weakness and age-related frailty appear related, at least in part, to low levels of vitamin D. Of course, weak muscles can reduce energy and activity levels. A deficiency of vitamin D levels may increase someone's susceptibility to getting colds, the flu, and chronic infections, which are also causes of fatigue.

A lack of vitamin D has also been linked to depression and seasonal affective disorder (SAD). SAD is a type of depression that develops during the winter, when days are shorter and people are less likely to receive enough sunlight. Sunlight is needed to stimulate the body's production of vitamin D. Depression is a common cause of fatigue and lethargy.

B-Complex Vitamins

Several of the eleven B-complex vitamins play crucial roles in the burning of glucose and fat for energy. For example, vitamins B_2 (riboflavin) and B_3 (niacin) are the core molecules in compounds involved in energy production. Similarly, vitamin B_1 (thiamin) is needed to make specific enzymes that help break down carbohydrates. Processed carbohydrates (again, think in terms of breads, muffins, pastas, and sugary foods) contain little, if any, vitamin B_1, but they create a greater demand for these enzymes.

A lack of these B vitamins can cause a wide variety of symptoms, including low energy levels, depression, migraine headaches, sensitivity to stress, and delusions in some people. In particular, a lack of vitamin B_{12}, or a difficulty in absorbing it, can result in fatigue and weakness. Seniors have the greatest risk of vitamin B_{12} deficiency because they are more likely to suffer from atrophic gastritis, the inability to produce sufficient stomach acid. Acid-blocking drugs, which are among the most widely used over-the-counter and prescription medications, also reduce vitamin B_{12} absorption.

Iron-Deficiency Anemia

In the 1950s and the 1960s, iron-rich supplements were hyped as cures for "iron-poor tired blood." Because iron is an essential nutrient in mitochondrial energy production, a deficiency can in fact cause fatigue. Menstruating women have the greatest risk of developing iron deficiency, but too much iron in supplements can increase the risk of heart disease in men, postmenopausal women, and people with an iron-storage disorder, such as hemochromatosis. Therefore, take iron supplements only after a doctor has measured your blood levels and found them to be low.

If your blood levels of iron remain low after supplementing, you may have celiac disease, which can significantly reduce iron absorption. Celiac disease is essentially an allergy to gluten, a protein found in wheat, rye, and barley. If you are diagnosed with celiac disease, the only treatment is avoidance of foods that contain these grains.

Your Best Energy Foods: Protein and Vegetables

One of the greatest ironies regarding nutrition is that people rarely recognize the foods that will provide them with the most energy. These foods include quality protein and high-fiber vegetables, along with small amounts of minimally processed carbohydrates and oils tailored to each person's weight and activity levels.

The idea that protein is an energy food may be contrary to everything you have probably heard. Indeed, most of the controversies around protein have little to do with nutrition, and protein has acquired an undeserved negative reputation. Why such negativity? One reason is that high-protein diets have been criticized for being high in saturated fat. Yet depending on the specific food choices, high-protein and protein-centered diets can actually be low in saturated fat. Another reason is that many people view the consumption of animal foods (that is, protein) as being politically incorrect. The truth of the matter is that the word *protein* comes from the Greek word *proteios*, which means "first and foremost." Protein is fundamentally important to our health and to our energy levels.

Protein has also suffered from what might be called a public relations problem: many people feel that protein-rich foods are boring, that they aren't nearly as exciting to eat as pizza or pasta. A lack of excitement over protein, however, is often really a reflection of how protein and vegetables are prepared. A dry, overcooked piece of fish or chicken

> ### *quick tip*
> ### Handy Back-Up Foods for Energy
>
> You might think that it's just too difficult to rely on protein for an energy boost, but it's actually quite easy. Keep some deli turkey and cheese, along with mustard, handy in your refrigerator at home or the office. If you work out of your car, you can keep these in a cooler. Lay a slice of turkey over the cheese, drizzle a little mustard down the middle, and pinch it like a taco. Use apple slices as a side.

won't be very appealing, but you have probably eaten some truly memorable protein-centered meals, such as a tasty steak, a piece of rotisserie chicken, or broiled seafood. (I'll describe my approach to food and recipes later in the book.)

The bottom line? Protein is essential for maintaining stable energy levels. I recommend that you include some protein with breakfast, lunch, and dinner so that your energy remains steady all day long.

Protein and High-Fiber Vegetables Stabilize Blood Sugar

Your optimal blood sugar level falls within a fairly narrow range, and your energy and mental concentration decrease when your blood sugar either rises too high or sinks too low. (The healthiest blood sugar range is between 75 to 85 mg/dl, and 79 to 80 mg/dl appears to be optimal.) Oscillations in your energy levels usually reflect extreme shifts in blood sugar, which are often the consequence of eating sugar and other types of processed carbohydrates. As I discussed earlier, people who always feel tired tend to have elevated blood sugar levels, and those who experience up-and-down peaks and troughs in their energy during the day often have sharp fluctuations in their blood sugar levels.

In contrast to sugars and starches, eating protein usually does not produce extreme changes in blood sugar. Over a period of days and months, a moderate-to-high protein diet will actually reduce and normalize blood sugar levels if they have been elevated. (This "null effect" is why protein-rich foods, such as fish, poultry, and meats, are rarely mentioned in lists that describe the glycemic index of foods.) By stabilizing blood sugar levels, protein helps puts an end to frequent up-and-down energy fluctuations during the day. Protein also stabilizes blood sugar by moderating the blood sugar spike of any carbohydrates you consume at the same meal.

High-fiber vegetables—almost any veggie except potato—have a similar stabilizing effect on blood sugar, particularly when the vegetables are consumed raw or lightly cooked (as in sautéed or steamed, so that they're still a little crisp and not mushy). In high-fiber vegetables, the carbohydrate remains part of a fibrous matrix, and this fiber slows or blocks the digestion of the carbohydrates. A combination of protein and high-fiber vegetables is ideal: your two most important food groups.

You don't have to consume a lot of protein to improve your blood sugar or your energy levels, in case you're concerned about being on a high-protein diet. Essentially, you'll be replacing many of the carbs in your diet with protein or vegetables, and those vegetables (again, with the exception of potatoes) will contain high-quality carbohydrates. For breakfast, one egg and some high-fiber fruit (such as raspberries, blueberries, or kiwifruit) should suffice. A bowl of steel-cut oatmeal will have a beneficial effect on blood sugar similar to that of protein; instant oatmeal will not. For lunch, consider a chicken Caesar salad (minus the croutons) or another salad that includes some protein (for example, tuna). For dinner, a piece of fish or poultry roughly the size of the palm of your hand should be sufficient, with twice the quantity of vegetables.

Protein Preserves and Increases Muscle

Your skeletal muscles—that is, the muscle groups of your arms and legs—are the body's primary engine for burning food for energy. Protein is essential for making muscle; after all, muscle consists of protein. Biochemists consider protein to be the workhorse of the body because it is needed to make hormones, enzymes, and the structure of our skin and internal organs. Sugars and other carbohydrates create fat, not muscle.

As people get older, they lose skeletal muscle and may even develop a muscle-wasting condition known as sarcopenia. This loss of muscle increases frailty, impairs balance, and contributes to prediabetes. Studies have shown that eating more protein or taking amino acid supplements—amino acids being the building blocks of protein—actually increases muscle and carbohydrate tolerance in seniors, even without exercise.

The risk of sarcopenia, however, doesn't begin at age sixty-five. You sow the seeds of either strong or weak muscles throughout your life. As a general rule, the more muscle you can maintain as you age, the more energetic and physically independent you will be.

Animal Protein Provides Mitochondria

Animal protein, specifically muscle meats (e.g., beef, lamb, or dark chicken and turkey), is usually very dense in mitochondria. We can't use these mitochondria, per se, but we can use the mitochondrial nutrients (for example, L-carnitine and CoQ10) they contain to support our own mitochondria and energy-generating processes. The richest source of mitochondria and mitochondrial nutrients is actually organ meats, such as the heart and the liver, which were once routinely used in cooking but are rarely eaten anymore.

Many people unknowingly deprive themselves of rich sources of mitochondrial nutrients. For example, they prefer white chicken or turkey breast meat, which is high in protein but relatively low in mitochondria. The legs and the thighs, which are more muscular, have higher concentrations of mitochondria. The color of those darker meats is actually related to their concentrations of iron-rich mitochondria.

Green vegetables, such as dark lettuce, spinach, and kale, contain chloroplasts, which are the plant equivalent of mitochondria. Chloroplasts convert the energy of sunlight into specific energy-generating compounds, such as B vitamins, ATP (adenosine triphosphate), and

NADP (nicotinamide adenine dinucleotide phosphate, which is related to vitamin B_3). These same compounds play essential roles in our energy production, so eating vegetables also helps feed our own mitochondria.

Nutritionally Dense Foods Are the Keys to a Healthy Diet

One of the best ways to evaluate the quality of foods is to think in terms of their nutrient density. Sugars and sugarlike carbohydrates have a lot of calories, but they do not contain many vitamins and minerals or other nutrients. In contrast, protein and vegetables are nutrient dense—they have a diversity of nutrients that are important to your health. High-quality protein sources, such as fish, chicken, turkey, and eggs, provide vitamins, minerals, amino acids, and healthy fats but very little saturated fat. Most vegetables also contain vitamins and minerals, along with large amounts of dietary fiber.

Another way of looking at nutrient density is to think about the nutritional value of every bite or calorie of food that you consume. An ice cream cone and a piece of salmon may have the same number of calories, but which one is more nutritious? Eating for nutrient density provides your body with high-quality nutrition. In contrast, sugars and carbohydrates contain very few nutrients.

The diet of ancient humans—essentially, what the human race grew up eating—consisted primarily of animal protein and a wide assortment of plant foods. These are our best, most nutrient-dense energy foods. High-starch and high-sugar foods did not become part of our diet until the advent of agriculture about ten thousand years ago and even more so over the past fifty years. Some anthropologists have pointed out that the consumption of grain-based starches (and most processed sugars are made from grains) led to the sudden appearance of arthritis, birth defects, and other health problems. Human genes have not yet adapted to the large amount of dietary sugars and carbohydrates that people now consume.

Starchy foods did have value when our ancestors worked hard physically. Now, with so many people being sedentary and overweight, it's obvious that we consume too many nutrient-weak foods. It only makes sense to reduce our intake of sugar and starch calories and to return to some semblance of our ancient and healthier eating habits. This doesn't mean we have to live like cavemen and cavewomen or eat exactly the way they did, but improving our eating habits is imperative if we want to maintain overall health, lose weight, and to enhance our energy levels.

The Importance of Water

Many people overlook the importance of hydration—that is, of consuming sufficient amounts of water throughout the day—in promoting overall health and in energy. Dehydration, or poor hydration, from drinking low-quality beverages is a problem among all age groups and particularly among seniors, who often forget to consume liquids. Most of your body consists of water, and dehydration leads to reduced biochemical activity and to your organs becoming smaller in size. Brain shrinkage, which is usually a factor in dementia, appears strongly related to the inadequate consumption of fluids over many years.

Life on Earth has depended on water for millions of years. It is still essential for our health. Quite simply, water is a key ingredient in the chemistry of life and energy. (Each molecule of water consists of two atoms of hydrogen and one atom of oxygen, and both elements play important roles in energy production.) When we tamper too much with the water we consume, we alter the chemistry of the body. For example, thirst is the body's way of indicating a need for water, but many people attempt to quench that thirst with a soft drink, juice, or beer. The body is asking for water, but we give it a calorie-packed liquid.

Like protein, water has suffered from a serious public relations problem—people tend to think it's boring and the drink of last resort. There are actually many healthy and tasty forms of water that can contribute to hydration and other aspects of health. Mineral water, especially European brands (for example, Perrier, San Pellegrino, Gerolsteiner, and Blu), contain substantial amounts of calcium and magnesium, which help the body produce energy. A squeeze of lemon or lime juice adds flavor to any glass of water. In addition, Ayala's herbal waters and Hint flavored waters contain herb and fruit essences for flavoring, but without any calories.

Many types of tea offer an alternative to coffee and water. Most herbal teas do not contain any caffeine, although you must read labels carefully to avoid added sweeteners. Green and black teas typically contain less caffeine than coffee does, and, depending on the brand, they may contain substantial amounts of L-theanine, which, as I've noted, counteracts the negative effects of caffeine in the tea.

Nor do you have to drink all of the water you consume. Vegetables and fruits contain substantial amounts of water, which contribute to your overall hydration. I discourage the regular consumption of most juices, however, because they contain too much sugar, sometimes more than soft drinks do. I make an exception for coconut water, sold in 11-ounce containers. You can drink one per day. Although coconut water contains a small amount of naturally occurring sugars, it is one of the richest sources of dietary potassium (approximately 660 mg per 11 ounces).

High-Energy Eating Habits

In addition to a diet that emphasizes protein and high-fiber vegetables, I also recommend specific eating habits to enhance and help maintain high energy levels. I discuss eating habits in chapter 7.

The Importance of Breakfast

Breakfast was once a staple of the American diet. Yet during the last thirty years, the practice of eating a full breakfast has largely disappeared for many different reasons, including a lack of time and, frequently, the desire to skip a meal to lose weight. Skipping or skimping on breakfast is no longer a uniquely American problem. In cities around the world, people have told me that lack of time forces entire families to leave home for work or school with nothing more than a cup of coffee, a glass of milk, and something sweet.

Skipping breakfast leads to high blood sugar, insulin, and adrenal hormone levels, all of which ultimately contribute to people feeling tired. Having a bowl of cereal, a fruit smoothie, an energy bar, or a doughnut or another pastry (essentially, a dessert) isn't any better. Such habits set the stage for a midmorning blood sugar crash, and ironically, breakfast skippers end up eating more during the rest of the day and gaining more weight, compared with people who do eat breakfast. In one study, women who ate a sugar- and carb-rich breakfast (compared with women who ate eggs) ended up consuming an extra 400 calories during the following day and a half—the equivalent of thirty pounds of calories in the course of a year.

Eating a protein-centered breakfast can have a near-immediate and impressive effect on your energy levels. For example, almost all of the clients I coach on nutrition had a habit of skipping or skimping on breakfast when they first came to see me. Over and over again, they reported a dramatic improvement in their energy levels on the first morning that they ate a protein-rich breakfast. Their energy increased and remained steady at least through noon, and most found that they did not desire a large lunch. Because they ended up eating less, losing weight became almost effortless.

Aaron's Health and Energy Levels Improve with Better Eating Habits

Aaron, who was in his late twenties, had been wrestling with a number of health concerns, including elevated levels of blood fats, moderately high blood sugar, and low energy levels. He started following my dietary advice—the program in *Stop Prediabetes Now* and *No More Fatigue*—and had impressive improvements within the first month.

His total cholesterol decreased from 320 mg/dl to 188 mg/dl, and his low-density lipoprotein (LDL) dropped from 230 mg/dl to 118 mg/dl. In addition, his triglycerides went from 188 mg/dl to 58 mg/dl and fasting glucose from 101 mg/dl to 80 mg/dl.

These were all significant improvements indicating a much lower risk of heart disease and diabetes. But Aaron also felt a lot better. He stopped feeling "wiped out" after meals, and his indigestion, bloating, and other symptoms related to irritable bowel syndrome went away.

Making the Time to Eat Healthier Meals

You may think that eating breakfast is fine in theory, but that few people actually have the time. Many individuals skip breakfast because they are too rushed in the morning. Yet the reason they don't have time is that they were too tired to get up early enough to make and eat breakfast. It becomes a self-perpetuating loop, in which one act causes the next. This is a common situation, with caffeine affecting their sleep quality and excess sugar causing persistent feelings of tiredness.

Eating a protein-centered breakfast can help you maintain your energy as you reduce your caffeine consumption. Protein will also diminish your cravings for sweets. In addition, protein will help you feel less stressed during the day, in large part because the amino acids that compose protein help promote a more stable brain chemistry and moods.

Try my time-saving breakfast tip. The idea is to make the time that you invest in preparing one breakfast pay off for three breakfasts.

On a Sunday morning, sauté some onions, bell peppers, and mushrooms (or vegetables of your choice), and add scrambled eggs, a little cooked brown rice, and some grated cheese. Make the equivalent of three breakfasts, using three to six eggs. Eat one-third of the scrambled eggs that morning and store the rest in wrapped bowls in the refrigerator, heating each one in a microwave oven on Monday and Tuesday. On Wednesday morning, cook steel-cut oatmeal—it will take about thirty minutes, so you can start it before you get into the shower or make it the night before. Have one bowl of oatmeal that morning (add raspberries, blueberries, and powdered cinnamon for flavor), and refrigerate and then reheat the extra servings of oatmeal. On another morning, have a light and quick breakfast consisting of a few slices or pieces of turkey or chicken and cheese with some fresh fruit.

Cultivate consistent meals and snack times. It is important to maintain relatively consistent meal and snack times. When we feel stressed, such as by deadlines or having too many things to do, we tend to delay or skip lunch—until our blood sugar drops and we become irritable or we physically crash. As I've already noted, some sort of sweet or junk food is not the healthiest solution. I recommend keeping healthier food handy. This could include cheese, deli turkey, and an apple in the refrigerator. You can also make your own trail mix (an assortment of nuts) and pack it in small plastic bags for a healthy midafternoon snack. This way, you can avoid the candy and the chocolate that are added to many commercial trail mixes.

Avoid late-night or off-hour snacking. Researchers have long known that night-shift workers have a greater-than-average propensity for gaining weight. It turns out that working late hours can alter one's eating habits. In addition, according to studies conducted at Northwestern University in Evanston, Illinois, eating at the "wrong" times can affect normal circadian rhythms, change circadian-dependent gene behavior, increase weight, and lead to less physical activity.

Eat smaller portions. Dinner plates and meals are bigger today than they were fifty years ago, and, not surprisingly, people on average consume several hundred more calories daily than in the past. Overeating is a major reason why people are tired. Sometimes they feel so stuffed after a meal that they express regret after getting seconds or eating that extra piece of pizza. Having smaller portions doesn't mean you have to starve yourself. Gain control of your meal size simply by skipping seconds. Then aim to reduce your portions by 10 to 20 percent. It's not that difficult—you'll feel a lot better, and you will have more energy after the meal.

In the next chapter, I discuss the third circle of fatigue, to show how shifting hormone levels can affect your energy levels.

chapter 3

Hormones and Fatigue

Chronic stress, poor dietary habits, and biological changes in middle age can set the stage for low levels of several hormones, which will result in feelings of persistent tiredness and contribute to the Fatigue Syndrome. Sometimes younger people will also be affected by significant changes in hormone levels.

Hormone issues form the third circle of fatigue. In this chapter, I focus primarily on how adrenal exhaustion and hypothyroidism (low thyroid activity) can cause fatigue. I will also touch on how low levels of estrogen and progesterone in women and declining testosterone in both women and men can contribute to fatigue.

Several different hormone problems may overlap in the Fatigue Syndrome, and careful medical testing may be needed to determine the primary hormonal problem. Correcting hormonal imbalances usually requires a combination of nutritional support (because vitamins, minerals, and proteins are needed to make hormones) and natural bioidentical hormone-replacement therapies. Some hormones are available over the counter at health food stores, whereas others will require a physician's prescription. Either way, I urge you to work with a physician to accurately diagnosis low hormone levels and to monitor your treatment. Please do not attempt to self-treat suspected hormone problems with either over-the-counter or prescription hormones (such as those you might borrow from a friend or a family member).

Adrenal Exhaustion

Have you dealt with chronic stress for many years—for example, by juggling work and parenthood—and now you feel totally exhausted and ready to crash whenever you stop? Or have you become so dependent on coffee that it's essential for sharpening your reflexes and mind in the morning and to keep you going throughout the day? If your answer to either question is yes, there is a good chance that you're approaching or already suffering from adrenal exhaustion.

Adrenal exhaustion is known by a number of names, including adrenal burnout, adrenal fatigue, and adrenal insufficiency. It is a disease of our modern stress-filled lives, in which we try to do too much in too little time and don't allow sufficient space in our schedules for relaxation, restful sleep, and eating healthy foods. Sometimes it can be difficult to distinguish between the symptoms of adrenal burnout and those of low thyroid. If you happen to suffer from both, you and your physician must treat your adrenal burnout first. There are two reasons for this: sometimes low thyroid function is a consequence of adrenal exhaustion, and without treating the adrenal exhaustion first, thyroid hormone medications can aggravate adrenal stress (that is, the lead up to adrenal exhaustion).

The adrenals are small hormone-secreting glands located atop each of your kidneys. They serve as your stress-response glands and release a variety of hormones to maintain homeostasis—biological balance—in response to stresses. The best known of these hormones are adrenaline (your fight-or-flight hormone) and cortisol (your long-term stress hormone). When faced with chronic stress, your body shifts from making adrenaline to cortisol. Adrenal burnout occurs when you lose your ability to make cortisol, which leads to exhaustion and fatigue.

Some of the most common symptoms of adrenal burnout include tiredness, weakness, listlessness, caffeine cravings, and orthostatic hypotension (low blood pressure and lightheadedness when standing up). A variety of gastrointestinal symptoms can also point to adrenal fatigue, such as gastritis, abdominal cramps, nausea, and vomiting. In addition, salt cravings, sugar cravings, feeling unusually cold, pollen allergies, and food and chemical sensitivities can be signs of adrenal burnout.

Just because you feel totally exhausted, however, doesn't mean that you suffer from adrenal burnout. James L. Wilson, N.D., D.C., the author of *Adrenal Fatigue: The 21st Century Stress Syndrome*, has noted a common pattern that is characteristic of adrenal burnout: A person will wake up feeling tired even after sleeping for eight or more hours. He or she doesn't feel completely awake until later in the morning or until after consuming caffeine. Energy levels dip during the afternoon, but the person gets a second wind at around 6 p.m. or 11 p.m., then doesn't feel tired enough for sleep until later.

Unfortunately, many physicians will not make a formal diagnosis of adrenal exhaustion except in cases of Addison's disease, also known as primary adrenal insufficiency, which is the most severe form of the disorder. Nearly all of the symptoms of Addison's disease and other (secondary) types of adrenal insufficiency are identical, with the exception of one: people with Addison's disease have hyperpigmentation of the skin, which may be most evident in a darker color of the skin, especially underneath the fingernails and in darkened creases in the palms of the hands.

---

quick tip
The Link between Caffeine and Adrenal Burnout

Did you recently have to increase the amount of coffee (or an energy drink) you consume just to get going in the morning or to keep going during the day? A sudden and sustained need for more caffeine can be a clue to adrenal burnout.

The Origins of Modern Stress Theory and Adrenal Exhaustion

The word *stress*, as we use it today, was coined in the 1930s by Hans Selye, M.D. An expert in hormones, Selye developed a concept of "general adaptation syndrome" to explain how people and animals physically adapt to stress. Selye's ideas became widely popular in the 1950s after he wrote *The Stress of Life* (McGraw-Hill, 1956).

Alarm, the first stage of chronic stress, is characterized by enlarged adrenal glands, a surge of adrenal hormones, and reduced immunity. The second stage, that of resistance (or adaptation), is marked by chronically elevated cortisol levels. During the second stage, a person appears to be functioning normally, but it is the unusually high levels of cortisol that maintain the apparent adaptation to stress. It is impossible for a person to indefinitely adapt to major stresses without serious consequences occurring, however, so after months or years, the adrenals' ability to secrete large amounts of cortisol starts to falter. That leads into the third stage, exhaustion, which is characterized by the inability to continue adapting and the appearance of adrenal exhaustion symptoms. Signs of damage to the adrenal glands may or may not be apparent in this final stage.

Selye's three stages of stress might initially sound a bit abstract. To make them more tangible, consider a soldier entering a war zone. During his first combat experience, his body responds with a surge of adrenaline. As the soldier stays in the war zone, living with a day-to-day fear of being attacked and killed, his body adapts by producing large amounts of cortisol. When his body can no longer maintain that level of cortisol production and adaptation, he slips into the exhaustion stage, which might be diagnosed as post-traumatic stress disorder (PTSD), instead of adrenal exhaustion. PTSD is also common among caregivers and crime victims; once it was called "a nervous breakdown."

The Causes and the Progression of Adrenal Burnout

Any and all types of stress can contribute to adrenal fatigue, and the more stresses you have in your life, the greater your risk of eventually developing adrenal burnout. Stress forces your adrenal glands to work harder to shield your body against those pressures. Poor eating habits contribute to adrenal burnout, because junk foods do not supply the nutrients you need to support adrenal hormone production.

Cortisol-inducing stresses include deadlines at work, unpleasant bosses and coworkers, relationship difficulties, financial worries, negative attitudes, irritability, and anger. Staying up late night after night, not getting enough sleep, and not having sufficient "down time" can add to the stress. So can smoking tobacco, consuming too much caffeine, and having allergies and repeated infections. The biggest life stresses are the death of a spouse and divorce, and these can also lead to adrenal exhaustion.

Many illnesses and medications can increase the chances of developing adrenal exhaustion. Diabetes, rheumatoid arthritis, Crohn's disease, allergies, *Candida* (yeast) infection, and hepatitis are often intertwined with adrenal exhaustion, either as a contributing factor or as a consequence. The continuous use of oral, topical, and intranasal glucocorticoid (cortisone-containing) drugs, such as prednisone, can suppress normal adrenal function. So can antifungal drugs and some anticoagulants, such as warfarin and heparin. Consuming grapefruit juice can increase the potency of these drugs, because the juice suppresses activity of the liver enzyme CYP3A4, which normally breaks down many medications. Low sodium levels (hyponatremia) and dehydration are also potential causes of adrenal exhaustion.

Long-term, abnormally high levels of cortisol accelerate the aging process and depress production of dehydroepiandrosterone (DHEA), which is often regarded as an antiaging hormone. In fact, a high-cortisol, low-DHEA pattern may indicate that a person is heading toward adrenal burnout. You need DHEA to make estrogen, progesterone, and testosterone, so high cortisol levels can interfere with your sexual hormones and libido. Cortisol can also impair the body's production of the active form of thyroid hormone, so chronic stress can have far-reaching effects.

Still more health problems can stem from too much cortisol. The hormone increases blood sugar levels and the "bad" low-density lipoprotein (LDL) form of cholesterol, which boosts the risk of developing type 2 diabetes and coronary heart disease. Combined with high levels of insulin, cortisol promotes the formation of fat around the belly. Although abdominal obesity is usually considered a dietary problem, it is also related to stress.

All of these negative effects of cortisol, however, are merely the prelude to adrenal burnout. Chronically elevated levels of cortisol are not healthy, but it is low levels of cortisol that characterize adrenal exhaustion, in which the body's defenses collapse.

If you have adrenal exhaustion, it is important to improve your adrenal function as soon as possible. In addition to leaving you feeling tired much of the time, untreated adrenal exhaustion can make you more susceptible to frequent and chronic infections, including those involved in chronic fatigue syndrome, and it may also increase your long-term risk of developing cancer.

Adrenal Exhaustion Was at the Root of Nicole's Fatigue

Nicole, at age fifty-five, was looking forward to retiring in the next several years. She had worked most of her life as a hospital nurse but recently found herself increasingly dependent on coffee to have enough energy to get through the day. In addition to fatigue, she experienced low blood pressure, occasional dizziness, less stamina, and aches in her arms and legs.

She consulted a nutritionally oriented physician, who ordered some tests and diagnosed her with adrenal insufficiency, although it was not severe enough to be Addison's disease. The doctor suggested that she make some dietary changes, liberally add salt to her foods, and take several vitamin and herbal supplements. After several weeks, Nicole found that her energy was returning. After four months, all of her symptoms, including the aches, had disappeared.

Assessing Your Risk of Adrenal Burnout

Many signs and symptoms point to adrenal burnout. If you check five or more items on the following lists, you may have it or be at risk. If that's the case, it may be worthwhile for you to undergo more formal testing.

Top Five Signs of Adrenal Burnout

- ☐ Fatigue (excessive)
- ☐ Dizziness when standing up quickly (orthostatic hypotension)
- ☐ Hypoglycemia (frequent periods of low blood sugar)
- ☐ Mood problems (such as depression, poor concentration)
- ☐ Aches or pain in the muscles of the upper back, the arms, and the neck

Other Signs of Adrenal Burnout

- ☐ Abdominal pain
- ☐ Alcohol intolerance
- ☐ Allergies
- ☐ Anorexia
- ☐ Autoimmune diseases (for example, rheumatoid arthritis)
- ☐ *Candida* (yeast) infection
- ☐ Coffee cravings (more than two cups daily)
- ☐ Concentration (poor)
- ☐ Confusion (occasional)
- ☐ Cravings for sweet foods
- ☐ Dark skin pigmentation (under the fingernails and in creases in the palms of the hands)
- ☐ Depression
- ☐ Diarrhea and constipation (alternating)
- ☐ Feeling unusually or atypically cold
- ☐ Fear (feelings of)
- ☐ Fingernails (brittle or with ridges)
- ☐ Frustration (feelings of)
- ☐ Gastrointestinal problems
- ☐ Glucocorticoid drug use (chronic)
- ☐ Hair loss (unexplained)
- ☐ Headaches
- ☐ Heart palpitations

(continued)

Other Signs of Adrenal Burnout (*continued*)

- [ ] High-carb, low-protein diet
- [ ] Hypotension (low blood pressure)
- [ ] Illness (chronic)
- [ ] Inflammatory diseases
- [ ] Indigestion
- [ ] Irritability
- [ ] Lightheadedness
- [ ] Low body temperature
- [ ] Major life stress (death of a spouse, divorce, or loss of a job in the last year)
- [ ] Memory (poor)
- [ ] Overexercise
- [ ] Overwork
- [ ] Premenstrual tension
- [ ] Salt cravings
- [ ] Skin (dry or thin)
- [ ] Sleep (inadequate)
- [ ] Staying up late at night
- [ ] Stress (chronic)
- [ ] Surgery
- [ ] Too much to do (feelings of)
- [ ] Weak muscles or difficulty increasing muscle mass
- [ ] Weight (difficulty gaining)

Getting Your Cortisol Levels Tested

Most conventional physicians will try to assess adrenal function with a single blood test to measure either cortisol or a provocative test for cosyntropin or ACTH (adrenocorticotropic hormone) levels. These tests are notoriously inaccurate, however, except in the more serious cases of adrenal exhaustion. If your doctor relies only on these blood tests, he may assume that you are not suffering from adrenal burnout.

To measure your cortisol levels, I recommend that you get a cortisol saliva test. The test kit, which your doctor can order from Diagnos-Techs (diagnostechs.com), involves providing four saliva samples on a typical day, which you do at home or at work by saturating four cotton wads with saliva. You provide the saliva samples between 7 a.m. and 8 a.m., noon and 1 p.m., 4 p.m. and 5 p.m., and 11 p.m. and midnight. This approach minimizes the error of relying on results from a single blood test, which does not reflect normal cortisol variations during the course of a day. As a general rule, cortisol levels tend to be highest in the early morning and to decline steadily during the day and the evening. In addition, a saliva test can measure your cortisol/DHEA ratio.

Treatments for Adrenal Burnout

Restoring normal adrenal function takes time, an average of four months to one year, and typically involves modifying your lifestyle, improving your diet, taking nutritional supplements, and possibly using medications. It is essential that you be certain that you have adrenal burnout before you follow my recommendations.

First, you must modify your daily habits to reduce the impact of stress and so that you get sufficient restful sleep. (See chapter 10 for ways to improve your sleep.) Many people benefit from psychological counseling to lessen their "reactive" response to stress. One technique is to cultivate a psychological "reset button," which I describe in chapter 9, to help you recognize when you feel too stressed.

Second, you can support normal adrenal function by adopting a diet that emphasizes good-quality protein and high-fiber vegetables

---

quick tip
Sugar and Salt Cravings

Cravings for either sweet or salty foods may be a sign of adrenal stress and adrenal exhaustion. Sweet foods will quickly raise blood sugar levels, offsetting the hypoglycemia that is often associated with adrenal exhaustion. Approximately one in five people with low blood levels of sodium has secondary adrenal exhaustion, and salt cravings are an attempt to boost sodium levels.

and minimizes unnecessary refined sugars, refined carbohydrates, and junk foods. Yet your style of eating is just as important as the food itself—in particular, you should have slower, more enjoyable meals, instead of wolfing down fast foods. (See chapter 7 for specific dietary recommendations.)

Third, you must either wean yourself off coffee or reduce the amount of caffeine you consume in coffee, tea, and soft drinks. Doing so will improve your restful sleep, which is crucial to bouncing back from adrenal exhaustion. As you recover from adrenal exhaustion, you will become less dependent on coffee to prop yourself up, so reducing coffee consumption will be easier than you might expect. Please refer back to chapter 2 for my suggestions on how to reduce caffeine dependence, as well as to chapter 10 for advice on improving sleep.

Fourth, a number of nutritional supplements can be extremely helpful in dealing with both adrenal stress and adrenal exhaustion. Vitamin C and pantothenic acid (a B vitamin) play especially important roles in the body's manufacture of adrenal hormones.

Supplements for Both Adrenal Stress and Adrenal Exhaustion

I recommend starting with a high-potency multivitamin supplement that contains 50 to 75 mg each of vitamins B_1, B_2, and B_3. There are many high-quality supplements on the market, but I like the Carlson (carlsonlabs.com) and Solgar (solgar.com) brands, which are sold in health food stores.

Next, add extra amounts of the following supplements to enhance your adrenal function:

- *Vitamin C*   Take at least 1,000 mg three times daily. Too much vitamin C will loosen your stools, so if that happens, simply reduce the amount.
- *Pantothenic acid*   Take approximately 500 mg twice daily of this B vitamin, in addition to the amount that is in your multivitamin.

In addition, consider adding these supplements, as well:

- *Phosphatidyl serine*   Take 500 mg twice daily with food.
- *Zinc*   Take 15 mg twice daily with food.
- *N-acetylcysteine*   Take 500 mg of this antioxidant twice daily.

Supplements That Help in Adrenal Exhaustion

If you suffer from adrenal exhaustion, you can use several herbs to help restore normal adrenal function. Of these herbs, licorice is the most important.

- *Licorice root*   Take licorice root supplements, but be sure to use a product that is not deglycyrrhizinated. Deglycyrrhizination removes the active compound (glycyrrhetinic acid) that inhibits the breakdown of cortisol. You can buy nondeglycyrrhizinated licorice root tinctures from Nature's Answer (naturesanswer. com) and Oregon Wild Harvest (oregonwildharvest.com). I also like Solgar's Deglycyrrhized Licorice Root Extract because it contains both deglycyrrhized licorice and raw licorice root. Follow the label directions for using these products. Do not eat licorice candy because it contains sugars, and many of these candies are not actually made from licorice. *Note*: Large amounts of nondeglycyrrhizinated licorice may cause hypertension, so consider monitoring your blood pressure.
- *Rhodiola rosea*   This herb is considered an adaptogen, meaning that it helps you adapt to stress. It improves adrenal function. Take 200 to 300 mg daily.
- *Siberian ginseng*   Siberian ginseng (*Eleutherococus senticosus*) is also an adaptogen. Take 200 to 300 mg daily.
- *Ashwagandha* (*Withania somnifera*)   Ashwagandha can be helpful as well. Take 500 mg daily.

You can buy most of these herbal supplements in the Solgar or Nature's Way brands, which are sold at most health or natural food stores. A good combination supplement is Natural Factors AdrenaSense (naturalfactors.com), which contains rhodiola, Siberian ginseng, ashwagandha, and other herbs, but not licorice.

In addition, people with adrenal burnout need to liberally salt their food, which will help counter low blood pressure. For this purpose, I recommend two brands of natural salt, Celtic Sea Salt (celticseasalt.com) and RealSalt (realsalt.com), which are sold in health food stores and are available on the Internet. Because both licorice root and salt can increase blood pressure, do monitor your blood pressure. As your symptoms of adrenal exhaustion improve, you will want to be careful not to develop high blood pressure.

Other Treatments for Adrenal Burnout

Assuming that adrenal burnout has been confirmed by laboratory tests, you and your physician might consider adding an adrenal-hormone supplement. IsoCort, manufactured by Bezwecken, contains freeze-dried porcine adrenal cortex and is available from numerous Web sites without a prescription. Although IsoCort can be purchased without a prescription, do not take it without a physician's guidance! (Many naturopathic physicians, compared with allopathic physicians, are more familiar with treating adrenal exhaustion.) Take three tablets of IsoCort on waking and three more at noon, unless your doctor suggests a different dosage. You can increase the absorption of IsoCort by allowing the small tablets to dissolve under the tongue instead of swallowing them. Another excellent product is Terry Naturally's Adrenaplex (europharmausa.com), which contains freeze-dried adrenal extract, licorice root, small amounts of pregnenolone and dehydroepiandrosterone (both are over-the-counter hormones), and several other ingredients.

Nutritionally oriented and alternative physicians may prescribe low doses of hydrocortisone as part of a broader regimen to restore normal adrenal function. Low-dose hydrocortisone is very different from more powerful steroid and cortisone-family drugs (such as prednisone), and it rarely causes side effects. The typical protocol is to take four 5 mg hydrocortisone tablets daily (one with each meal and one at bedtime with a light snack). This dose is 1/60th to 1/300th that of high-dose prednisone, which can cause serious side effects.

Another option is to take 25 to 50 mg of dehydroepiandrosterone (DHEA) daily, according to a report in the *New England Journal of Medicine*. The physician-author of the article suggested DHEA for patients with adrenal exhaustion whose sense of well-being and physical strength is below normal, as well as for patients with depression. Again, do not take DHEA without a clear diagnosis of adrenal exhaustion and a physician's guidance.

As you recover from adrenal exhaustion, you will notice that your symptoms gradually improve. For example, you will feel less tired, have fewer episodes of dizziness, and fewer muscle aches; you will likely experience fewer caffeine cravings.

Barb's Psychological Problems Turned Out to Be Adrenal Exhaustion

Physicians attributed Barb's extreme fatigue, low-grade fever of unknown cause, sleep disorders, and loss of weight, despite high calorie intake, to emotional and mental disorders. But Barb knew her health problems were real and physical, and antidepressant medications provided no benefits.

Finally, tests at a nutritionally oriented medical clinic found that Barb was actually suffering from adrenal exhaustion, and that the cognitive effects of her sleep deprivation and extreme weight loss had likely been misdiagnosed as depression. Barb's cortisol levels were extremely low, except at bedtime, which probably contributed to an abnormal circadian rhythm. Normally, cortisol levels are highest in the morning and lowest at night.

Barb's treatment program included a high-protein diet, plus B vitamins to correct deficiencies, as well as medications to help restore her cortisol levels. Although her progress was slow, it was steady, and Barb now feels much better than before.

Low Thyroid Activity

Your thyroid hormones regulate your metabolism—that is, your body's ability to burn carbohydrates and fats for energy and to generate body heat. We may not be cold-blooded reptiles, but our energy levels and body temperature often go hand in hand. We also need thyroid hormones for normal development of bone, muscle, and the brain.

Fatigue is one of the most common symptoms of low thyroid activity, or hypothyroidism, and it affects a higher percentage of middle-age women than men. Other common symptoms include unexplained pain, dry skin, and brittle or ridged fingernails. Low levels of thyroid hormones may also be associated with an unexplained weight gain, hair loss (particularly the eyebrows), irritability, depression, an inability to sweat, and cold hands and feet. Assuming that you have considered adrenal burnout as a cause of your fatigue, the next step is to investigate whether you might have low thyroid activity.

Considerable research indicates that low thyroid activity is common in people who are overweight. In other words, some people really do have slower metabolisms. This doesn't mean that correcting low thyroid will lead to weight loss, and you should never take thyroid medications with weight loss as an objective. Because low thyroid activity interferes with normal carbohydrate and fat metabolism, it can worsen glucose control in people with type 2 diabetes. One study found that about one in every twenty patients with type 2 diabetes had low thyroid activity, but the prevalence of hypothyroidism was one in ten among women with diabetes.

Nutrition and Your Thyroid Gland

Nutrition has a very strong bearing on your thyroid hormone levels. The thyroid gland, located in your neck, secretes two principal hormones: T4 (thyroxine) and T3 (triiodothyronine). Both hormones are made from the amino acid L-tyrosine (found in protein) and iodine. T4 has four iodine atoms. Enzymes called deiodinases convert T4 to T3, which has three iodine atoms and four times the hormonal activity of T4. Iodine is an essential dietary nutrient, and if you don't get enough of it from either your diet or supplements, you cannot make adequate amounts of thyroid hormones.

The pituitary gland responds to iodine deficiency by secreting large amounts of thyroid-stimulating hormone (TSH), which may eventually enlarge the thyroid in an effort to scoop up more iodine from the bloodstream. Iodized salt contains extremely small amounts of iodine, enough to prevent a grossly enlarged thyroid gland (goiter), but not enough to provide other benefits to the thyroid gland. If you have low levels of selenium, another essential nutrient, this can complicate the picture. You need selenium to make deiodinase enzymes, so inadequate selenium in the body impedes the conversion of T4 to T3.

Hypothyroidism is far more common than an overactive thyroid gland, and the most commonly diagnosed form of low thyroid is an autoimmune disease called Hashimoto's thyroiditis, in which the body's immune cells attack the gland. Forty percent of people with chronic fatigue syndrome (CFS) have Hashimoto's thyroiditis. Hypothyroidism is also very common among people with fibromyalgia. The more common problem, however, may actually be subclinical hypothyroidism, in which the symptoms of low thyroid activity are less obvious.

Determining Your Thyroid Activity

Low thyroid activity can cause a variety of physical and behavioral symptoms. If you check five or more items on the following lists, you may have, or be at risk of developing, hypothyroidism. The odds of having low thyroid activity increase with the number of symptoms you check. To confirm the diagnosis, take your basal body temperature and then ask your physician to measure your blood levels of three hormones: TSH, T4, and T3.

Top Five Signs of Low Thyroid Activity
- ☐ Fatigue
- ☐ Headaches

(*continued*)

Top Five Signs of Low Thyroid Activity (*continued*)
- [ ] Cold hands and/or feet
- [ ] Constipation
- [ ] Depression (unexplained)

Other Signs of Low Thyroid Activity
- [ ] Acid indigestion
- [ ] Acne
- [ ] Allergies
- [ ] Anxiety
- [ ] Arthritis/achy joints
- [ ] Asthma
- [ ] Bad breath
- [ ] Blood pressure (low)
- [ ] Bruising
- [ ] Caffeine use (increased)
- [ ] Carpal tunnel syndrome
- [ ] Cholesterol (elevated)
- [ ] Cold intolerance
- [ ] Colds and sore throats (frequent)
- [ ] Constipation
- [ ] Concentration (poor)
- [ ] Coordination (poor)
- [ ] Eyebrows (loss or thinning)
- [ ] Eyes (dry or blurred vision)
- [ ] Falling asleep during the day
- [ ] Exhaustion
- [ ] Fluid retention (edema)
- [ ] Flushing of skin
- [ ] Gastric reflux
- [ ] Hair (dry, loss, or prematurely gray)
- [ ] Hives
- [ ] Hypoglycemia
- [ ] Infertility
- [ ] Insomnia

- ☐ Irritability
- ☐ Irritable bowel syndrome
- ☐ Itchiness
- ☐ Lightheaded feeling
- ☐ Low motivation
- ☐ Memory (poor)
- ☐ Menstrual cramps
- ☐ Menstrual periods (irregular)
- ☐ Migraines
- ☐ Muscular aches
- ☐ Nails (unhealthy looking)
- ☐ Panic attacks
- ☐ Premenstrual syndrome
- ☐ Ringing in the ears
- ☐ Self-esteem (low)
- ☐ Sexual development inhibited
- ☐ Sex drive (reduced)
- ☐ Skin (dry)
- ☐ Skin infections (increased)
- ☐ Skin pigmentation (changes)
- ☐ Sweating (lack of)
- ☐ Throat (abnormal swallowing sensations)
- ☐ Tiredness after eating
- ☐ Tobacco use (increased)
- ☐ Ulcers
- ☐ Urinary infections (frequent)
- ☐ Weight gain (unexplained)
- ☐ Wound healing (slow)
- ☐ Yeast infections (frequent)

Measuring Your Basal Temperature

In addition to completing the checklist, you can measure your "basal temperature," which is your body temperature when you wake up but before you get out of bed. Once you move around, your body temperature will rise, and you won't be able to accurately take your basal temperature.

To do this test, you'll need an old-fashioned oral glass thermometer, which you can buy at most drugstores. Shake the thermometer down before you go to bed, and leave it within easy reach. As soon as you wake up, while moving as little as possible, place the thermometer in the fold of your skin in your armpit, and leave it there for ten minutes. Write down the temperature, and repeat this for three consecutive days. If you are a woman, do not take your basal temperature during your menstrual period or on the day when you think you will be ovulating—your temperature will be slightly higher at those times.

A normal basal temperature will be between 97.8 and 98.2 degrees Fahrenheit. If your basal temperature is 97.7 degrees or lower, you are likely hypothyroid. A temperature above 98.2 degrees might be suggestive of either an infection or hyperthyroidism.

If you believe you are hypothyroid, based on the checklist and/or on your basal temperature, ask your physician to measure your TSH, free T4, and free T3 levels. It is essential that your doctor measure all three, because measuring only TSH or T4 will not detect subclinical hypothyroidism. These are the results you need to pay attention to:

- If your TSH level is elevated, even if it is in the high-normal range, you likely have low thyroid activity. High TSH points to hypothyroidism, even if T4 and T3 levels happen to be normal.
- If your TSH and T4 levels are normal, but your T3 is low or low-normal, you probably have difficulty converting T4 to T3. Low or low-normal T3 is a common sign of subclinical hypothyroidism.

It may initially be difficult to interpret your T4 and T3 numbers, in part because medical laboratories use three different scales (pmol/L, ng/dL, pg/dL, and pg/mL) to present their test results. Complicating the situation, most physicians are far more familiar with T4 than with T3 activity, so they have a bias toward looking only at T4 levels. Ask your doctor for a copy of the report—don't accept his saying, "Everything is normal."

Here's how to make sense of your test results: In all cases, the blood-test report will note your specific blood level of T4 and T3, plus the "normal" range. If your T4 level is in the middle or high part of the range, that's good. If your T4 is either low or in the low-normal range, it is too low. Your T3 level should be in a comparable place in the range; if it is low or in the low-normal range, it is probably too low.

For example, let's say that your free T4 is 1.5 ng/dL (out of a range of 0.8 to 1.7 ng/dL), which means your T4 is high normal. If your T3 is 2.6 ng/dl (out of a range of 2.4 to 4.2 pg/mL), it is low normal, indicating poor conversion of T4 to T3. This is significant because T3 is the most active type of thyroid hormone.

Thyroid Hormone Relieves Liz's Depression

Liz is a successful painter, and her artwork is in collections around the world. Yet for twenty years she wrestled with depression. Both natural (Saint-John's-wort) and pharmaceutical (Prozac) treatments were not successful in relieving her deep feelings of depression.

Through all of this, Liz suspected that her depression was related to low levels of thyroid hormones. After all, she had other symptoms suggestive of hypothyroidism, such as unexplained weight gain, hair loss, and not sweating (even though she lived in the desert). Because blood tests showed her thyroid hormone levels to be in the normal range, doctors refused to give her a trial prescription of thyroid hormones.

Finally, when Liz was in her early fifties, she found a physician who was willing to prescribe thyroid medication for her to try. Twenty minutes after taking the first pill, Liz began to sweat. It was a vindication that she had been right about her self-diagnosis all along. Within a couple of weeks, her symptoms of depression vanished, and her husband and friends now describe her as being "effervescent."

Ways to Treat Low Thyroid Activity

You can correct low thyroid activity with a combination of natural thyroid extract and nutritional supplements. You'll need the help of a nutritionally oriented physician or at least a doctor who is open-minded enough to fully listen and respond in a supportive way to your concerns about hypothyroidism. Almost everyone feels better when his or her T4 and T3 levels move from low- to mid-normal to high normal.

Most physicians will prescribe one of several forms of synthetic T4 (levothyroxin, such as Synthroid, Levoxyl, or Levothroid) for low thyroid. Although synthetic T4 can help many people, it is of no benefit for those who have difficulty converting T4 to T3. People fare much better by taking Armour Thyroid (also sold as Westhroid and Nature-throid), a natural form of the hormone that is obtained from desiccated porcine thyroid glands. Armour Thyroid is standardized to provide a four-to-one ratio of T4 to T3. Because T3 has four times the activity of T4, this thyroid extract provides therapeutically equivalent amounts of T3 and T4. Armour Thyroid also contains tiny amounts of T1 and T2, which are found in our bodies, but their functions are not well understood.

You may have to give your physician some guidance in prescribing Armour Thyroid, because he or she will likely be more familiar with the dosing of synthetic T4. That's because medical school and drug company sales staffs emphasize T4 over T3. (A conversion calculator is available at www.armourthyroid.com/hcp_treatment .aspx#Armour.) In general, it is best to start at one of the lower dosages of Armour Thyroid, such as ¼ grain (15 mg) or ½ grain (30 mg) daily. Your doctor should consider increasing the dosage by ½ to 1 grain (60 mg) every two to three weeks until you achieve a desirable improvement in symptoms. The online calculator is also helpful if you want to switch from a synthetic to a natural thyroid product. *Caution*: Any sign of heart irregularities, such as angina pain or a racing heartbeat, indicates that the dose is too high and should be immediately reduced, regardless of whether the thyroid medication is natural or synthetic.

Two other forms of T3 are available by prescription, although I do not think they are quite as effective as Armour Thyroid. Thyrolar is a synthetic combination of T4 and T3 with a ratio comparable to that of Armour Thyroid. This is a reasonable choice for people who do not want to consume a porcine-derived product because of religious or ethical reasons or because of food sensitivities. Another option is Cytomel, a synthetic form of T3.

Nutritional Support for the Thyroid Gland

Nutritional support of thyroid hormone production is crucial. The three key nutrients are L-tyrosine (an amino acid or protein building block), iodine, and selenium. L-tyrosine forms the chemical foundation of thyroid hormones, as well as of adrenaline and dopamine—basically, the body's natural uppers. I recommend taking 500 mg of L-tyrosine immediately on waking, about ten to fifteen minutes before you consume any food or liquid other than water. You can take larger amounts if your physician thinks they would be helpful. *Contraindication*: If you have hypertension, monitor your high blood pressure after taking L-tyrosine because it may increase blood pressure. Stop taking L-tyrosine if you have an unsafe increase in blood pressure.

Iodine forms part of T4 and T3, but most iodine supplements are of such low potency that they provide little benefit. Likewise, the amount of iodine in kelp supplements is too low to have a significant thyroid-boosting effect. A better supplement is Iodoral, which contains 12.5 mg (12,500 mcg) of iodine in the form of 5 mg of iodine and 7.5 mg of potassium iodide. It is available from many different sources (such as celticseasalt.com) without a prescription. I recommend taking one-half to one tablet each morning. Take iodine supplements with food. Another useful product is Terry Naturally Thyroid Care (europharmausa.com), which contains 30 mg of iodine and 400 mg of L-tyrosine per each two-capsule recommended dose. This dose of iodine may be unnecessarily high (unless recommended by a physician), so I suggest just one capsule daily.

Selenium is crucial for converting T4 to T3, and people with hypothyroid will benefit from 200 to 400 mcg of this mineral daily. A study conducted at the U.S. Department of Agriculture's research center in Grand Forks, North Dakota, found that taking 200 mcg of supplemental selenium increased T3 levels in men and T4 levels in women during a two-year period.

Selenium is found in most multivitamin/multimineral supplements, so you may already be getting enough of it. Do not exceed 400 mcg daily without guidance from your physician. Take selenium supplements with food, but check the labels on other supplements (such as multivitamins) you might be taking, because they may already provide this amount of selenium.

Finally, it is important to restate the importance of correcting adrenal burnout (if it is present) before you start to take any prescription form of thyroid hormone medication. High levels of cortisol interfere with the conversion of T4 to T3, leading instead to the production of "reverse T3." Reverse T3 does not function as a real thyroid hormone. Instead, it attaches to cell receptors for T3 and blocks the activity of T3.

---

quick tip
Working with Your Physician

Many physicians understand that patients now have access to medical information on the Internet and want to be involved in their diagnosis and treatment decisions. Yet some people have told me that their physicians remain old-fashioned and close-minded and simply refuse to order tests for both T4 and T3.

It's important to remember that your physician works for you—and it sometimes helps if you tactfully remind your doctor of this fact. If your doctor is "old school" and dismisses your concerns about more comprehensive thyroid (or adrenal) testing or borderline low results, let him know in a matter-of-fact way that his lack of cooperation is not acceptable. Don't yell at him, but do explain your expectations of the physician-patient relationship. If he still refuses to, let's say, order tests for both T4 and T3 (instead of for only T4), let him know that you have no choice but to find another physician—and then do so. There is no reason to put up with mediocre medical care. You will likely have more cooperation from a naturopathic (N.D.) physician, although you will probably have to pay out of pocket for some of his services.

Testosterone Helps Michelle Regain Her Energy

Michelle was a high-energy corporate executive when, at age forty-eight, she felt as though she "hit the wall." Her boundless energy suddenly seemed to evaporate.

She went to the doctor expecting to find that her estrogen levels were decreasing, but tests determined that low estrogen was not the problem. Rather, her testosterone levels were far below normal for a woman her age. Michelle's doctor prescribed a small testosterone patch, and within a couple of weeks, her former energy levels returned.

Estrogen, Progesterone, Testosterone, and Insulin

Most of us have learned that estrogen and progesterone are "female hormones" and that testosterone is the "male hormone." It may surprise you to learn that healthy women and men secrete all of these hormones. Estrogen and progesterone are the principal sexual hormones in women, but women also make small amounts of testosterone. Testosterone and other androgens are the principal hormones in men, but men normally make trace amounts of estrogen.

Around age fifty, however, women experience several hormonal shifts. During perimenopause, estrogen and progesterone production decreases substantially, with the most common symptoms being hot flashes and lower energy levels. Perimenopausal symptoms may be more intense in women who have had a history of estrogen dominance—that is, being prodigious producers of estrogen but weak producers of progesterone, which moderates the effects of estrogen. Women with estrogen dominance usually have had a history of premenstrual syndrome, endometriosis, uterine fibroid tumors, or fibrocystic breasts.

Physicians who treat women for perimenopause tend to focus on estrogen and progesterone (in part, because of pharmaceutical company marketing) and overlook the possible roles of low adrenal or thyroid hormones, as well as elevated insulin levels, in midlife health issues. Oftentimes, there is a clustering of hormone issues in the Fatigue Syndrome. High insulin levels are indicative of insulin resistance, one of the signs of prediabetes and type 2 diabetes, and fatigue is a common symptom. It takes more time and effort to investigate and treat individual patients, instead of routinely (and all too casually) writing prescriptions for estrogen and progesterone.

Conventional hormone-replacement therapy relies on one type of estrogen, estradiol, which eases or eliminates hot flashes and other perimenopausal symptoms. After thirty years of aggressive pharmaceutical industry marketing and advertising, however, researchers found that estradiol significantly increases the risk of developing breast cancer and coronary artery disease. Bioidentical hormone replacement, which is considered an alternative and more natural therapy, appears to achieve the same benefits with fewer long-term risks. Bioidentical hormone replacement therapy often emphasizes estriol, a noncarcinogenic form of estrogen. Likewise, bioidentical progesterone is similar to the progesterone that women naturally secrete, compared with synthetic forms of the hormone, and it can help correct estrogen dominance in both premenopausal and perimenopausal women.

With hormone levels in play during middle age, some women also experience a decline in testosterone. Two symptoms are commonly suggestive of low testosterone levels in women: low energy and reduced libido. Making a correct diagnosis can be tricky, especially if there is an overlap of adrenal burnout, hypothyroidism, and prediabetic elevations in insulin levels.

If medical tests confirm low testosterone levels, bioidentical testosterone can usually relieve the fatigue. Testosterone can also reinvigorate a woman's sexual desire. In one study, reported in the *New England Journal of Medicine*, researchers used testosterone to treat postmenopausal women with low libido. None of the women, who were in their midfifties, were taking estrogen. The testosterone heightened the women's libido and led to a greater number of what the researchers described as "satisfying sexual episodes." The most common negative side effect was an increased growth of facial hair.

Although testosterone production can decline suddenly in men, it is more common for levels to decrease slowly over many years. Some-

> ### quick tip
> ## The Link between Estrogen and Vitamin D
>
> The effects of low vitamin D, which is needed to maintain strong bones, are amplified by declining levels of estrogen, according to research presented at a 2009 meeting of the American Heart Association. It's very possible that the bone-building benefits of estrogen-replacement therapy are due to its increasing the activity of vitamin D. The vitamin is also safe, whereas conventional hormone-replacement therapy poses serious risks.
>
> As we get older, our biochemistry becomes less efficient. We have greater difficulty breaking down food into its individual nutritional constituents and using those nutrients to make hormones. Yet any therapy will be more effective when it is combined with good nutrition and eating habits. Conventional physicians routinely ignore the nutritional building blocks of our hormones. For a great many reasons, I recommend that people with declining hormone levels take a high-potency multivitamin/ multimineral supplement and also a multi–amino acid supplement. These two supplements provide key nutritional support for the manufacture of our hormones.

times the problem is not testosterone production per se, but an abnormal surge in estrogen (which is made in the testes, the adrenal glands, or the abdominal fat cells). This increase in estrogen in men may be related to a greater activity of aromatase, the enzyme that converts testosterone to estrogen in both men and women. If you are a middle-age man and your energy or libido is in a slump, ask your physician to measure both your testosterone and aromatase levels. If your aromatase is elevated, the best natural treatment is supplemental chrysin, an antioxidant flavonoid found in plants. Chrysin inhibits the formation of aromatase.

The problem with estrogen and testosterone therapies is that they can increase the risk of cancer in both women and men. For this reason, it is important to assess this risk as best as possible, particularly of women developing hormone-dependent breast and ovarian cancer and men getting prostate cancer, before beginning to take these hormones.

chapter 4

Illness and Fatigue

Your lifestyle, eating habits, and hormone levels influence your long-term risk of developing serious chronic diseases, the fourth circle of fatigue. Fatigue is a primary symptom of many diseases, including chronic fatigue syndrome, fibromyalgia, multiple sclerosis, cancer, and the most serious forms of heart disease. Furthermore, many of the medical treatments for these diseases can exacerbate feelings of fatigue. For example, surgery, chemotherapy, and radiation take a heavy toll on the energy levels of cancer patients. Even commonly prescribed medications, such as cholesterol-lowering statins and antidepressants, can cause muscle weakness and fatigue.

Unfortunately, space precludes me from discussing the role of fatigue in every disease and treatment. Instead, I will explain several key principles that show how fatigue is intertwined in serious diseases, and then I will address the role of fatigue in various common chronic diseases and medical treatments. Some of these diseases involve impaired mitochondrial function, which interferes with the body's ability to break down foods for energy. This link to mitochondrial activity suggests potential nutritional and therapeutic approaches to help resolve the problem.

The Role of Inflammation in Fatigue

Inflammation occurs in every disease process. Sometimes it is a cause and other times an undercurrent in the disease. Inflammation is needed to fight infections and stimulate the healing process, but chronic inflammation is not normal. It is a sign that something is awry, and chronic low-grade inflammation significantly increases the risk of heart attack, stroke, Alzheimer's disease, and many other serious health problems.

What many people don't understand is that pro-inflammatory cytokines—part of a family of chemicals produced by the body—can cause fatigue. For example, pollen allergies can intensify feelings of tiredness, and this is partly the result of high cytokine levels. Food allergies can also boost cytokine levels, so inflammation is likely a factor in fatigue that occurs after meals.

Cytokines signal the cells to increase or decrease inflammation, so they set in motion a wide range of biological responses. The most problematic cytokines are tumor necrosis factor alpha, interleukin-1, interleukin-6, and C-reactive protein. These and other pro-inflammatory cytokines tend to be abnormally elevated in people who have various types of fatigue, including chronic fatigue syndrome and fibromyalgia. Studies have shown that pro-inflammatory cytokines multiply in people who undergo cancer treatments, such as with radiation. High levels of cytokines also interfere with the conversion of thyroid hormone T4 to T3, leading to low thyroid activity.

You can reduce inflammation levels in your body by cutting down on sugars and refined carbohydrates or eliminating them from your diet and consuming only sugars and carbohydrates that are naturally found in vegetables and fruits. Certain nutritional supplements are also very helpful in alleviating inflammation, such as the omega-3 fish oils, gamma-linolenic acid (GLA, a plant oil), vitamin D, curcumin (an extract of turmeric root), and Pycnogenol (French maritime pine bark extract). I recommend Carlson's Inflammation Balance supplement, which contains the omega-3s, GLA, and vitamin D. Another of my favorite remedies is Solgar's Pycnogenol and Turmeric Root Extract. For more information on this important subject, please refer to my book *The Inflammation Syndrome*.

General Principles on the Link between Disease and Fatigue

Chronic degenerative diseases develop slowly, almost always taking ten to twenty years (or longer) before the symptoms become obvious enough for a specific diagnosis. Here are several areas to be aware of.

- Nutrients form the foundation of your biochemistry and tissues, and nutritional therapies (including dietary modifications and the use of supplements) can usually lead to significant improvements in health. Nutrients usually work more slowly than drugs do, however, in terms of reducing symptoms, but they are crucial for recovery, healing, and restoring your energy levels.

- Doctors, hospitals, and other health-care organizations provide little, if any, support for the healing process after surgery. This gap is especially serious after major surgery (such as for cancer, heart disease, or osteoarthritis). As a consequence, recovery times are much longer than they optimally could be, and some people never really bounce back from the stress of surgery. Exacerbating the situation, muscle weakness is a common side effect of long stays in hospital intensive care units.

- Drug therapies (ranging from aspirin to prescription drugs) can lead to a rapid reduction of symptoms, but without changing the underlying disease process. Treating symptoms is not the same as treating the actual causes of disease. For example, a recent study found that drugs that are used to lower blood sugar in people with diabetes did not reduce inflammation, so a major part of the disease process still caused damage. Despite an enormous medical pharmacopoeia—ten thousand prescription and a hundred thousand over-the-counter drugs—few drugs are truly considered cures for diseases.

■ Drug therapies often have side effects, and the more drugs you take, the greater your risk of having side effects, including fatigue. Often, the second or third (or subsequent) drugs are prescribed to counter the side effects of other drugs. Many commonly used drugs, such as antihistamines and cholesterol-lowering statins, can cause fatigue. The more medications you take, the more likely they will be a factor in your fatigue.

Chronic Fatigue Syndrome

Twenty years ago, many physicians considered chronic fatigue syndrome (CFS) a psychosomatic disease, a type of hypochondria. The condition's symptoms were often perplexing because there were no clear diagnostic criteria and no approved medical treatments for CFS. The chief symptoms consist of a profound and prolonged fatigue lasting for at least six months. Other symptoms commonly include abnormal or unusual immune-system responses, depression, insomnia, headaches, mental fuzziness, and exhaustion after relatively mild exertion, such as walking.

More than three thousand studies have since shown that CFS is a real disease, yet it can still be difficult to diagnose. The cluster of symptoms is often highly individualized, and many physicians make the diagnosis only after eliminating other possible diseases. Indeed, CFS often overlaps other diseases, and, according to the Centers for Disease Control and Prevention (CDC), somewhere between 35 and 70 percent of people with CFS also have fibromyalgia. The CDC estimates that at least one million Americans have CFS, although only 20 percent of them have been actually diagnosed. It tends to affect more women than men. CFS is typically diagnosed when people are in their forties, but the disease can develop at any age.

Causes of Chronic Fatigue Syndrome

There is no single cause of chronic fatigue syndrome (CFS), but several factors do seem to precipitate it. CFS has often been described as a flu that does not go away, and at least two viruses have been implicated, although, confoundingly, viral infection is not always associated with CFS.

Many people with CFS have reported developing their debilitating fatigue after contracting influenza or, at least, an influenza-like infection. The Epstein-Barr virus, which also causes mononucleosis, has frequently been implicated in CFS. Although teenagers generally recover fairly quickly from mononucleosis (nicknamed the "kissing disease" because of one route of transmission), the infection can be more debilitating for people in their thirties and forties. Doctors may test for antibodies to the Epstein-Barr virus as one way of establishing a CFS diagnosis. Sometimes, measures of Epstein-Barr viral concentrations are low, but that may be because the virus is in a dormancy phase, although the damage has already been done.

In 2009, researchers at the Whittemore Peterson Institute in Reno, Nevada, reported that two-thirds of people with CFS had signs of infection with the xenotropic murine leukemia virus-related virus (XMRV). In contrast, fewer than 4 percent of healthy people were infected with the XMRV retrovirus. Until the publication of this study, XMRV was considered largely a mouse virus, though it was also associated with the risk of prostate cancer in men. The research on XMRV does not clearly demonstrate cause and effect, but this virus might also be a contributing factor in chronic fatigue syndrome. However, the link between the XMRV and chronic fatigue remains controversial.

Another common precipitating event appears to be exposure to high levels of chemical toxins, such as pesticides or any number of industrial pollutants. In addition, some poisons, such as cadmium, cyanide, and arsenic compounds, directly interfere with the production of energy in mitochondria and may contribute to CFS. Trace amounts of these substances, found in pesticides and various industrial pollutants, could conceivably impair the body's ability to produce energy, even killing the person who was exposed. Cadmium is absorbed into the body when people smoke tobacco; it is also released into the air we breathe each time brakes are used in a car. Mining, smelting, and the burning of fossil fuels discharge arsenic into the environment, and the burning of rubber and plastic is a source of cyanide.

Clinical evidence suggests that adrenal exhaustion commonly precipitates CFS. A person who is run-down physically or psychologically is more susceptible to a wide range of viral infections, and adrenal exhaustion greatly impairs the body's ability to fight infections. People with adrenal exhaustion and CFS commonly have chemical and food sensitivities. Many people with CFS are extremely sensitive to odors and complain about perfumes and chlorine in water. Some people with CFS obsess about the foods they eat, because certain foods leave them feeling good and other foods make them worse.

CFS has psychological components as well. Long-term stresses, such as work deadlines and difficult relationships, seem to predispose people to the disease, although the link might actually be through adrenal exhaustion. In many cases, depression and not fatigue is the primary symptom. Many people with CFS strike others as being acutely sensitive to subtle changes in their bodies and health, often in an obsessive manner. They can also be overly sensitive to medications and react to them in unusual and negative ways. A report published in the *Archives of General Psychiatry* noted that people who had been emotionally and sexually abused in childhood were especially likely to develop CFS as adults. Any of these factors may also overlap in CFS.

Considering the many different causes, it is more than likely that a confluence of factors—viral infection, nutritional deficiencies, toxic exposures, and adrenal exhaustion—can combine in different ways to precipitate CFS. The specific combination of factors likely varies from person to person.

A Clear Diagnosis of CFS

According to the CDC, you should consider a diagnosis of CFS if two criteria are met.

1. The first criterion is unexplained and persistent fatigue unrelated to any type of ongoing physical exertion. This fatigue would be of recent onset, would not be relieved by rest, and would significantly reduce previous levels of activity.

2. The second criterion is the presence of four or more of the following symptoms for at least six months: impaired memory or concentration, extreme exhaustion after exertion, insomnia, muscle aches or pain, joint pain without swelling, headaches, frequent sore throats, or tender lymph nodes.

Ways to Increase Your Energy If You Have CFS

With CFS, the sooner you start a recovery plan, the more likely you will avoid years (if not a lifetime) of fatigue and other symptoms. I have seen people recover within several months of adopting such a program, although they do remain susceptible to stress, CFS flare-ups, and fatigue. It is important to have a physician evaluate you for adrenal exhaustion and low thyroid activity and, if necessary, to treat these conditions while also tackling CFS.

Adopting a protein-centered diet is paramount for people with CFS. Protein is rich in mitochondrial nutrients, and it stabilizes blood sugar, which helps you avoid fluctuating energy levels. It's also important to increase your intake of fiber-rich vegetables and fruits (which I discuss in more detail in chapter 7), while minimizing your consumption of sugars and very starchy foods.

Supplements of several nutrients that are involved in mitochondrial chemical reactions can also be of great benefit to people with CFS. These nutrients include coenzyme Q10 (200 mg daily), L-carnitine or acetyl-L-carnitine (1,000 to 3,000 mg daily), alpha-lipoic acid (200 to 600 mg daily), and ribose (2,000 to 4,000 mg daily). I also recommend a high-potency B-complex supplement because of these nutrients' diverse roles in energy production. Extra biotin (one of the B vitamins) may be particularly helpful—in the range of 3,000 to 5,000 mcg daily.

Multi–amino acid supplements can increase muscle density and prevent muscle wasting, a common occurrence in CFS. Under these circumstances, I recommend 10 grams daily of an amino acid blend containing eight to ten amino acids. In addition, some preliminary research suggests that quercetin (1,000 mg daily), an antioxidant found in onions and apple skins, stimulates the breakdown of food to energy and increases the number of mitochondria.

It is very important to find a nutritionally oriented physician (M.D. or N.D.) and to begin once or twice weekly infusions of intravenous vitamin C as soon as possible after the diagnosis of mononucleosis or CFS. These intravenous infusions should be continued for several months. High doses of vitamin C enhance immunity, improve the burning of dietary fats, and can prevent postinfection deficiency.

Although most people with CFS insist they do not have enough energy to exercise, it is crucial that they begin some type of daily physical activity regimen. Doing so will increase the number of muscle cells and mitochondria in those cells, as well as amplify the benefits of amino acid and quercetin supplements. It is only prudent, however, to begin such a program slowly to increase tolerance and avoid a relapse. A personal trainer would most likely be of benefit, but he should understand your physical limitations. Walking and using hand weights are excellent starting points.

Tad Recovers from Chronic Fatigue Syndrome

Tad was forty-two years old when his life came to a halt because of chronic fatigue syndrome (CFS). He had been working under constant deadlines at work, his marriage was breaking apart, and he frequently drank too much alcohol. After what he described as a debilitating flu in late 2007—a flu that completely sapped Tad's energy—doctors identified antibodies to a recent infection with the Epstein-Barr virus.

Tad was unable to work, had extreme difficulty concentrating and remembering, and slept twenty hours each day. Following the advice of several friends, he embraced a range of alternative therapies and began to take various nutritional supplements. He began doing Anjali restorative yoga (a type of guided meditation) and undergoing acupuncture treatments and osteopathic cranial-sacral therapy. At the same time, Tad started to take selenium, alpha-lipoic acid, carnitine, N-acetylcysteine, and omega-3 fish oils, as well as two supplements that have antiviral properties: L-lysine and olive leaf extract. He underwent ten intravenous infusions of high-dose vitamin C.

It's important to note that Tad stopped drinking alcohol and smoking marijuana. He also began to maintain a more balanced schedule and now goes to bed by 10:30 each night. He regained enough energy to return to work after three months. Otherwise minor colds may bring a return of his extreme fatigue, but his regimen and lifestyle now enable him to recover fairly quickly. "I'm hardly out of the woods yet and may never be completely," Tad said, but he has definitely avoided permanent debilitating fatigue.

Fibromyalgia

People with fibromyalgia share many of the symptoms of CFS, but the distinguishing characteristic of fibromyalgia is usually overwhelming musculoskeletal pain, rather than fatigue. A person with this disease will often say she has pain all over her body and that even a light touch on the skin exacerbates the pain. Other common symptoms include joint stiffness, depression, brain fog, moodiness, dry eyes and skin, and anxiety. Fibromyalgia is also associated with sleep problems, irritable bowel syndrome, headaches, facial pain, and sensitivity to odors and noises.

As with CFS, many physicians are frustrated by the difficulty of diagnosing and treating fibromyalgia. The complexity of the disease begs for a careful physical examination, laboratory tests, and individualized treatment. Officially, there is no known cause for the disease; however, infections, injuries in the spinal area, and preexisting sleep disorders seem to predispose some people to the disease. Most likely, the collection of symptoms known as fibromyalgia has causes that vary from person to person. The disease affects an estimated three to eight million Americans. Often, improvements are more incremental than dramatic.

How People with Fibromyalgia Can Reduce Pain and Increase Their Energy

Many symptoms of fibromyalgia point to nutritional deficiencies that conventional physicians routinely overlook and therefore remain untreated. As with CFS, a viral infection or some other type of immune or physical trauma could deplete nutrient reserves and impair energy production in mitochondria.

Several of the B vitamins—specifically, vitamins B_1, B_6, and B_{12}—have analgesic properties. It is very likely that an inadequate intake of these vitamins increases one's sensitivity to pain. Several studies acknowledge the pain-reducing effectiveness of B vitamins, and, in one study, moderately high doses of these vitamins (in combination) enabled patients to reduce the amount of pain-relieving drugs they needed after surgery.

Because people with low levels of vitamin D are more sensitive to pain, vitamin D supplements may help reduce pain as well. In one report, published in the *American Journal of the Medical Sciences*, researchers noted that vitamin D deficiency mimicked the symptoms of painful metastatic cancer. An article by doctors at a pain clinic noted that one-third of patients had marginal or deficient levels of vitamin D. Low levels of vitamin D have been linked to lower back pain, rheumatoid and other forms of arthritis, migraine, and neuropathy. A 2009 study published in *Endocrinology Practice* found that vitamin D supplements did in fact reduce fibromyalgia symptoms. Because vitamin D deficiency is common—affecting three of every four Americans—it is essential to ask your doctor to measure your blood levels of the vitamin. You may need to supplement in the range of 2,000 to 5,000 IU daily.

Acetyl-L-carnitine may be of particular benefit to people with fibromyalgia. Researchers at the University of Verona, Italy, gave patients a combination of 1,000 to 1,500 mg of oral acetyl-L-carnitine daily, plus a single injection of it (500 mg) over ten weeks. Fibromyalgia patients who received acetyl-L-carnitine had significant reductions in pain, compared with those who took placebos. The beneficial results were most likely the result of improved mitochondrial bioenergetics.

Some research also suggests that CoQ10 supplements might help people with fibromyalgia. Researchers have reported that fibromyalgia patients have an abnormal distribution of CoQ10 in their bodies. Another report found that taking a combination of 200 mg of CoQ10 and 200 mg of the herb ginkgo biloba extract for approximately three months led to a reduction in symptoms.

Pain is often a sign of inflammation, and several natural anti-inflammatory compounds may be helpful. The omega-3 fish oils contain eicosapentaenoic acid (EPA) and docosahexaenoic acid (DHA), which increase the body's production of prostaglandin E3, an anti-inflammatory hormone-like compound. Fish oils can be combined with supplements of gamma-linolenic acid (GLA), derived from borage seed, black currant, and evening primrose oils. GLA increases production of a complementary anti-inflammatory compound, prostaglandin E1. Both prostaglandin E1 and E3 suppress activity of prostaglandin E2, which is strongly pro-inflammatory. For fibromyalgia, I recommend 1,000 to 5,000 mg of fish oils containing EPA and DHA combined with 200 to 400 mg of GLA daily.

Finally, a study by doctors at the Mayo Clinic in Rochester, Minnesota, found that acupuncture led to a significant alleviation in fatigue and anxiety in fifty patients with fibromyalgia. The benefits were apparent after just one month. Related therapies, such as meditation, yoga, and stress reduction, might also be beneficial.

Cancer and Cancer Treatments

No other disease seems to arouse the visceral fear that is associated with cancer. The reason is that the diagnosis is intertwined with thoughts of extraordinary pain, wasting away, and greatly reduced life expectancy. Conventional treatments, such as surgery, chemotherapy, and radiation, often seem worse than the cancer itself. All too often, cancer patients, with their loss of weight and hair and their extreme fatigue, practically walk like ghosts.

That said, an estimated ten million or so Americans currently live with cancer, a number that includes people who were recently diagnosed and long-term survivors. In recent years, medical centers and pharmaceutical companies have tried to reposition cancer from being a terminal disease to a chronic treatable (though not curable) condition.

Nutrition Speeds Recovery from Surgery

A range of nutritional therapies can go a long way toward improving the prognosis of cancer patients and, even in the case of terminal patients, significantly enhancing overall quality of life during their remaining months. Although I will discuss some specific nutritional treatments—which are best used after a tumor has been surgically removed—I will focus more on ways of reversing the overwhelming fatigue that usually accompanies both cancer and its conventional treatments.

It is important to recognize that cancer patients are almost always deficient in multiple vitamins and minerals, yet conventional oncologists rarely measure blood levels of their patients' vitamins and minerals. Many of these deficiencies likely existed before the diagnosis of cancer and can be exacerbated by treatments and poor eating habits, including the low-quality meals provided to hospitalized patients.

Any nutritional deficiency will slow the healing process after surgery, which is usually the first type of treatment a cancer patient undergoes. Because of poor nutrition, most people do not adequately heal from surgery. In my opinion, it is practically criminal malpractice that doctors and hospitals ignore the role of fresh, healthy foods and nutritional supplements at this critical time. For example, many women undergo the removal of lymph nodes after breast cancer surgery, and as a result they have a high risk of developing lymphedema, an abnormal swelling of the arm as it fills with lymph fluid. Yet aggressive nutritional support following surgery can support healing and, I believe, reduce the risk of lymphedema.

Everyone needs vitamin C to make collagen, the most common type of protein in the body. Vitamin C has many other roles as well, such as supporting the immune system and helping in the manufacture of certain neurotransmitters. Surgery depletes the body's vitamin C reserves. One reason people tend to heal slowly after surgery and are susceptible to infections is that they are not getting nearly enough supplemental vitamin C. In one study, researchers calculated that surgical patients would require 1,150 mg of vitamin C daily to restore normal blood levels of the nutrients. This amount, while better than nothing, probably falls short of optimal postsurgical levels.

Undergoing surgery is profoundly stressful, as is anesthesia. (Nitrous oxide, one of the many anesthetic drugs used by doctors, wipes out the body's reserve of vitamin B_{12}, which is not replenished by nutritionally low-quality hospital diets.) Vitamin C is also needed to synthesize L-carnitine and other carnitine-containing compounds. Because these carnitine compounds help in the burning of fat for energy, inadequate vitamin C contributes to postsurgery fatigue.

High doses of vitamin C have therapeutic benefits in the treatment of cancer as well. When given intravenously in 50-gram or larger infusions, vitamin C exploits a weakness of cancer cells and increases the production of hydrogen peroxide, a generator of free radicals. Conventional doctors may scoff at the use of vitamin C as a nontoxic form of chemotherapy, but using free radicals to kill cancer cells is the same rationale that is behind both radiation and most chemotherapy treatments.

Large amounts of vitamin C also benefit terminal cancer patients. In a Korean study, researchers gave cancer patients a combination of intravenous and oral vitamin C. The patients responded with significant cognitive and emotional improvements, as well as better appetites. They experienced significant decreases in fatigue, pain, nausea, and vomiting. The doctors observed, "Improved health-related quality of life is important as much as a cure of cancer in terminally ill cancer patients who have an estimated survival of less than six months." If such a simple therapy helps people with terminal cancer, the benefits will likely be greater for those who are not in the last few months of their lives.

Improving Cancer Patients' Energy Levels

Many chemotherapeutic drugs damage mitochondria, setting the stage for fatigue, weakness, and heart failure. For this reason, some of the mitochondrial nutrients I've already mentioned can have a protective effect. Among these nutrients are CoQ10, L-carnitine, and alpha-lipoic acid.

L-carnitine may be of particular benefit in alleviating the fatigue caused by chemotherapy and radiation. Italian researchers gave supplements of L-carnitine to women who were undergoing treatments for cancers of the head and the neck, the breast, the ovary, the uterus, or the stomach. The regimen consisted of 2 grams of L-carnitine three times daily for four weeks. The L-carnitine supplements led to significant reductions in fatigue, improved appetites and muscle mass, and better overall quality of life.

The chemotherapeutic drug Adriamycin (doxorubicin) can damage the heart and cause heart failure, although sufficient supplemental CoQ10 will likely protect the heart without reducing the drug's effectiveness. CoQ10 almost always improves energy levels, and a series of case histories found that relatively large amounts (approximately 400 mg daily) led to the regression of breast cancers and reduced the recurrence of breast and liver cancers. In another study, adding CoQ10 to a conventional cancer treatment decreased the risk of recurrence.

Many conventional oncologists discourage their patients from taking any supplements while undergoing chemotherapy or radiation. Their reasoning is more theoretical than based on real biology. To explain, chemotherapy and radiation generate large numbers of free radicals to kill cancer cells, and antioxidants could conceivably reduce their effectiveness (because antioxidants neutralize free radicals). Yet several recent medical journal articles have shown that cancer patients taking high-dose antioxidants live longer, have less pain, and enjoy a higher quality of life compared with people who do not take supplements. Some of the studies show that antioxidant supplements actually enhance the effectiveness of chemotherapy and radiation.

Why are oncologists so down on antioxidants? It may be that oncologists don't understand that antioxidants do far more than simply neutralize free radicals. Antioxidants influence gene activity, strengthen the immune system (so that our bodies do a better job of fighting cancer), promote healing, and prompt cancer cells to self-destruct. In the treatment of individual patients and in a clinical trial, Jeanne Drisko, M.D., of the University of Kansas Medical Center, has demonstrated that combining intravenous vitamin C, high doses of oral antioxidants, and chemotherapy greatly improves survival in women with ovarian cancer, which generally has a poor prognosis. More than likely, the benefits of this integrative approach extend to other types of cancer.

It's important to note that small amounts of antioxidants aren't likely to be of benefit in cancer, and some research hints that low-dose supplements might even increase the risk of cancer recurrence. The key, then, is to opt for larger, rather than smaller, amounts if you choose to supplement. Again, check with a nutritionally oriented physician about any potential risks while you are undergoing chemotherapy or radiation. If you want to take a more conservative approach, you can wait until after radiation or chemotherapy to begin a high-dose supplement program.

Finally, it is important to note that the herb Saint-John's-wort can reduce the effectiveness of some chemo drugs so, again, check with your doctors if you are still undergoing chemotherapy. Saint-John's-wort increases the activity of a liver enzyme that is involved in breaking down chemotherapy drugs and other toxic compounds. In general, this enhancement of liver function is beneficial, but it may be problematic while you undergo chemotherapy.

One irony is that eating fruits and vegetables is frequently recommended to reduce the risk of developing cancer, but such nutrition suggestions are ignored once a cancer diagnosis has been made. Eating large amounts of produce provides an assortment of antioxidants and other nutrients. The one food with unclear benefits is grapefruit, which contains furanocoumarins, compounds that impede the activity of an essential liver enzyme. Because of this effect, grapefruit or grapefruit juice heightens the potency of many drugs, including statins, blood pressure medications, antihistamines, and antidepressants. There is some evidence suggesting that grapefruit might increase the risk of breast cancer, perhaps by suppressing the normal breakdown of chemicals in the liver.

Dealing with Chemo Brain

Up to 70 percent of cancer patients who undergo chemotherapy experience a type of mental fog called "chemo brain." Yet an animal study suggests that chemo brain can be prevented with supplements of N-acetylcysteine (NAC), an antioxidant. NAC is used in conventional medicine as the treatment for Tylenol overdose and to break down mucus in the lungs.

In the study, researchers at the West Virginia University School of Medicine, Morgantown, and their colleagues exposed laboratory rats to two commonly used chemotherapeutic drugs, Adriamycin and Cytoxan. The drugs interfered with the animals' memory; however, NAC prevented the animals' memory impairment. The dose of NAC was the human equivalent of 14,000 mg, a very large but safe amount. NAC is sold over the counter at most health food stores, and my hunch is that 5,000 mg daily might be adequate.

Preventing and Reversing Cachexia

One of the most worrisome aspects of cancer is cachexia (pronounced ka-kek'-see-uh), in which cancer patients lose large amounts of weight and muscle and literally waste away. The liver seems hell-bent on breaking down the body's muscle tissue to create glucose to feed the cancer cells. To some extent, cachexia results from pro-inflammatory molecules called cytokines, which the body produces in great quantities in response to the tumor.

Research studies have shown that cancer patients can take action to prevent or ameliorate cachexia. Following are some treatments that have proved successful.

Fish oil supplements To counter cachexia, doctors at the University of Iowa Carver College of Medicine, Iowa City, tested the effects of omega-3 fish oils, a natural anti-inflammatory. The body converts fish oils to prostaglandin E3, which dampens inflammation. Their subjects were forty-three advanced cancer patients who suffered from moderate to severe malnutrition. The patients each had lost an average of six pounds of body weight during the month prior to joining the study.

The doctors asked the patients to take a quantity of fish oil capsules relative to their weight. For example, a 154-pound person took eleven fish-oil capsules, adding up to 4.7 grams of eicosapentaenoic acid (EPA) and 2.8 grams of docosahexaenoic acid (DHA) daily, which are the biologically active constituents of fish oil. Because of their precarious health, only some of the patients were able to take the full amount of fish oils, but thirty-six of them took at least one capsule daily. During the next two to four months, twelve of the patients gained weight, ranging from about one-quarter pound to almost eight pounds, and six of these patients gained more than 5 percent of their body weight. Twenty-two lost weight, ranging from about one pound to thirteen pounds. Overall, patients lost an average of one and three-quarter pounds, a significant decrease from the start of the study. Although fish oils didn't help all of the patients, larger amounts given earlier would likely have resulted in greater resistance to cachexia.

Amino acid supplements   These building blocks of protein have been shown to increase muscle and stamina in seniors, and experimental evidence suggests that they can help prevent cachexia in cancer patients. One amino acid in particular, L-leucine, helps convert dietary protein to muscle. Other individual amino acids, however, including beta-alanine, L-ornithine, and combinations of amino acids, have helped increase muscle mass. I recommend taking 3 to 5 grams of a multi–amino acid supplement, containing three to ten amino acids.

Vitamin D   Cancer patients with cachexia suffer from both an increased rate of muscle breakdown and sluggish synthesis of new muscle. You need vitamin D to build strong bones and also to synthesize new muscle. Taking it won't give you the physique of a bodybuilder, but it will help your body make normal amounts of muscle protein. A large number of medical studies indicate that vitamin D helps prevent cancer, so it will likely improve your odds in fighting cancer as well. Vitamin D regulates the body's production of cathelicidin, a powerful immune compound that protects against cancer and infections. Vitamin D can also lessen pain.

Antioxidants This family of nutrients, which includes vitamins C and E, as well as many others found in vegetables and fruits, squelches harmful molecules called free radicals. This is important because free radicals fan the biochemical fires of inflammation. Cancer patients typically have abnormally high levels of free radicals (a state sometimes referred to as oxidative stress), and antioxidant supplements can often restore some semblance of balance and may help retard cachexia.

Heart Disease and Other Cardiovascular Diseases

Heart disease, stroke, and other blood-vessel diseases remain the leading cause of death for Americans and people in many other Western nations. Without question, advanced heart disease can result in debilitating fatigue, although it is usually intertwined with other serious health problems, such as obesity and chronic obstructive pulmonary disease. Yet the more immediate problem is this: widely prescribed drugs, particularly statin-class cholesterol-lowering drugs such as Lipitor, are a major cause of fatigue, muscle damage and weakness, and pain.

The roots of cardiovascular diseases amount to a medical tangle, in large part because of so many causative factors. Physicians routinely ignore the basic reasons why heart disease develops, namely, poor eating habits, overweight, and a lack of physical activity. Instead, they focus on symptomatic treatments, such as reducing cholesterol levels. Statins create an illusion of protection, while setting the stage for complacency and a panoply of short- and long-term side effects. Why bother eating healthier foods, losing weight, or exercising when a tiny pill will lower your cholesterol and supposedly solve everything? Not long ago, such miracle cures were dismissed as panaceas, but that was before the pharmaceutical industry began to spend billions of dollars each year to promote its drugs.

Coronary Artery Disease

Nearly everyone has heard that elevated blood levels of cholesterol are a cause of heart disease. Elevated cholesterol is certainly a sign that something is awry, but the evidence that cholesterol itself causes coronary heart disease is flimsy at best. (Calcium forms part of the fatty deposits that form in arteries, but we are not exhorted to consume less calcium!) At best, high cholesterol levels are nothing more than a modest indicator of risk, except in hereditary hypercholesterolemia. Half of all heart attacks occur in people with normal cholesterol levels, a fact that undermines the validity of high cholesterol levels as a way to predict a heart attack.

With such a hit-or-miss approach, measuring cholesterol levels is largely a waste of time. It's also a testament to medical faddism that millions of people have been talked into taking statins, and that medical groups periodically urge that millions more, including children, also take statins. Cholesterol is certainly easy to measure, and that ease has helped drug companies create enough worry to sell billions of dollars' worth of cholesterol-reducing drugs. Lipitor alone accounts for $13 billion in annual revenues for its maker, Pfizer, and it's only one of about a half-dozen statin drugs on the market.

Statins and Fatigue

The link between statins and fatigue lies in how these drugs work. Statins lower cholesterol levels by inhibiting an enzyme, hydroxymethyl-glutaryl-coenzyme A reductase (HMG-CoA reductase), which is needed for cholesterol production. Yet statins affect far more than cholesterol. All of the chemical reactions that depend on HMG-CoA reductase also get blocked by statins.

For example, your body uses HMG-CoA reductase to make CoQ10, which plays a fundamental role in energy production. CoQ10, which I've already discussed, is needed to complete a key step in the mitochondria's ability to produce energy. Without adequate CoQ10, these energy-generating chemical reactions cannot reach a climax.

Interfering with HMG-CoA reductase also inhibits the production of squalene, a compound that offers at least some protection against cancer. And if you consider that cholesterol is the core molecule in our steroid hormones—estrogen, progesterone, and testosterone—statins could have far-reaching negative effects on our health, energy, youthfulness, sexuality, and fertility.

The most common side effect of statins is myalgia, or muscle pain. By conventional medical estimates, myalgia and myopathy develop in 10 percent of statin users, but the actual number is probably higher. In a recent study of eighty-three patients, more than half suffered statin-induced muscle damage, including people who had stopped taking the drugs. That same study also found that the blood test (for creatine phosphokinase, or CPK) that doctors use to assess muscle damage from statins was essentially useless. According to some research, microscopic signs of muscle damage develop within days of taking statins. It is very possible that nearly everyone who takes a statin experiences some degree of muscle damage, which could take years to become clinically significant.

Rhabdomyolysis, which means a wasting away of muscle, occurs less frequently than myalgia, but it is far more serious. In rhabdomyolysis, muscle cells break down, and in the process we lose some of our ability to make energy. The symptoms of rhabdomyolysis range in severity, from mild to serious muscle pain and weakness, and may also include dark-colored urine. Statin-induced rhabdomyolysis is sometimes called "statin myopathy," meaning that the drugs have caused muscle disease. Statins can also reduce liver function, which may lead to fatty deposits in the liver, reduced glucose tolerance, and greater difficulty in breaking down toxins—all of which can also cause fatigue.

Typically, the most severe cases of rhabdomyolysis and impaired liver function raise medical red flags. Yet the repercussions from taking statins are not black and white: a person is not either well or having serious side effects. What happens is often much more subtle, with many individuals and physicians failing to recognize a connection between statins and fatigue. It's not that the drug companies are unaware of the risks of statins. Merck, which makes the statin drug Zocor, was granted two patents (numbers 4,929,437 and 4,933,165) for using CoQ10 in treating statin-related myopathies in 1990.

So, if measuring and treating elevated cholesterol is a dead end, what is a better risk factor to measure? In the late 1990s, Paul M. Ridker, M.D., and his colleagues at the Harvard Medical School found convincing evidence that chronic low-grade inflammation, not cholesterol, was a primary cause of coronary artery disease. They developed a test for high-sensitivity C-reactive protein (hsCRP) to measure this type of inflammation. Ridker found that people with elevated hsCRP levels were more than four times as likely to have a heart attack—a relationship far stronger than any risk associated with cholesterol. In a recent study of young men, doctors from the Geffen School of Medicine, Los Angeles, found that high levels of hsCRP were also closely related to feelings of fatigue in people in their thirties and forties.

Cardiomyopathy and Heart Failure

Just as the muscles of our arms and legs can break down in response to statins, so can the heart itself. After all, the heart is nothing more than a very specialized muscle with exceptional energy requirements to keep beating for seventy or more years.

Cardiomyopathy and heart failure have nothing to do with cholesterol levels and blockages in blood vessels. Rather, they describe a catastrophic loss of energy in the heart muscle, which reduces its ability to pump blood. The most common type of cardiomyopathy, called idiopathic dilated cardiomyopathy, means a disease of the heart muscle, an enlarged heart, and an unknown cause. The heart enlarges in an effort to collect and pump a greater volume of blood, but the heart's walls become thin and stiff—a type of muscle wasting. Cardiomyopathy and heart failure are the main justifications for heart-transplant surgery, which has a price tag of several hundred thousand dollars.

Talk with almost any cardiologist, and he or she will state that the prevalence of cardiomyopathy and heart failure has increased significantly during the last fifteen or so years. Indeed, cardiologists now see teenagers with cardiomyopathy, which until recently had been virtually unheard of in this age group. Both cardiomyopathy and heart failure cause extreme fatigue, poor circulation, and weakness after the slightest exertion. Untreated, cardiomyopathy will lead to congestive heart failure, meaning that fluids will settle into the lungs, leading to breathing difficulties.

Although statins increase the risk of cardiomyopathy and heart failure, there are other reasons for the greater prevalence of these diseases. One is that CoQ10 is virtually absent in the modern diet. As recently as fifty years ago, people commonly consumed large amounts of CoQ10 in organ meats, such as fried liver and heart and other giblets in turkey and chicken stuffing. These days, giblets are usually discarded. Because of the widespread consumption of junk foods since the 1950s, most diets in developed countries also lack appreciable amounts of the nutritional building blocks of CoQ10, so many people have difficulty making it on their own. In addition, some viruses specifically attack the heart muscle, damaging it and reducing its ability to pump blood.

CoQ10 supplements, however, when taken early enough and in sufficient amounts (typically, in the range of 300 to 400 mg daily), can reverse cardiomyopathy, heart failure, and some other types of heart diseases. Beginning in the 1970s, Japanese physicians began to use CoQ10 to treat cardiomyopathy and other forms of heart disease. In the early 1980s, the late Peter Langsjoen, M.D., of Tyler, Texas, directed the first U.S. clinical trials of CoQ10 in the treatment of heart failure. Incredibly, CoQ10 can often eliminate the need for heart transplants by reducing the severity of cardiomyopathy and heart failure.

Product Recommendations

Many nutrients benefit the heart, and I like the Nutra-Support Energy: Natural Fatigue Fighter formula made by Carlson Laboratories (carlsonlabs.com, 800–323–4141). It contains CoQ10, L-carnitine, alpha-lipoic acid, B-complex vitamins, and other nutrients. Most of the ingredients directly affect the ability of the heart to maintain its energy levels and output. Solgar (solgar.com), another excellent vitamin

> ## quick tip
> ### Many Drugs Can Cause Fatigue
>
> Chemotherapeutic drugs can cause profound fatigue, but they are not the only class of drugs that do so. Of the thousands of over-the-counter and prescription drugs on the market, almost five hundred are known to have fatigue as a possible side effect. Some of these drugs can continue to cause fatigue after a person stops taking them. Among the problematic medications are oral antibiotics, allergy drugs (including Claritin and Zyrtec), analgesics, antidepressants (such as Wellbutrin), antihistamines, benzodiazepines (for example, Valium), various heart and blood pressure drugs (including ACE inhibitors, beta-blockers, and statins), diuretics, sleep medications (for instance, Ambien), immune-suppressing drugs, and antiseizure medications (such as valproic acid).

company, sells many different potencies of CoQ10, liquid L-carnitine, and alpha-lipoic acid. I particularly like Solgar's 1,000 mg acetyl-L-carnitine tablets, and the company has a wide range of CoQ10 supplements, as well. Both the Carlson and Solgar brands are sold at most health and natural food stores.

Multiple Sclerosis, Autoimmunity, and Fatigue

Multiple sclerosis (MS) and other types of autoimmune diseases (including but not limited to lupus and rheumatoid arthritis) are common causes of fatigue. Many of these diseases share similar features, such as immune cells attacking the body's issues and inflammation-related fatigue. All of these diseases tend to be progressive, meaning they get worse over time.

In MS, immune cells attack the myelin sheaths that are wrapped around nerve fibers. *Sclerosis* is the medical term for "lesion," and in MS, scarlike lesions form on the myelin, which is somewhat like the plastic insulation around electrical wires. When the myelin becomes inflamed and deteriorates, it short-circuits nerve signals and leads to the disease's physical and neurological symptoms. Different MS symptoms are related to the locations of specific nerve damage, and those symptoms can take the form of extreme fatigue, weakness, a lack of balance, difficulty walking, double vision, speech problems, and depression. That's certainly bad enough, but the conventional treatment of MS involves immune-suppressing drugs, and fatigue is one of their side effects.

Often, medical and patient organizations state that the cause of MS (or other diseases) is unknown and that there is no cure, but such statements are disingenuous. The truth is that although there is rarely a single cause of MS, there are usually common factors leading up to the disease and accelerating its progression. Furthermore, while there may not be a "cure," numerous treatments can bring considerable relief and at least a partial reversal. Scientists may not yet understand all of the genetic, environmental, and molecular causes of MS, but the research does point to a cluster of biochemical and nutritional risk factors. Even if the link between a particular nutritional deficiency and a disease is scientifically fuzzy, it's hardly rocket science to recognize that nutritional deficiencies do not help anyone feel better.

Vitamin D   Researchers have long recognized that the incidence of MS is greater in populations that lie farther from the equator. The exception to this pattern is in regions or nations where people eat large amounts of fresh fatty fish, such as Japan. One common denominator between geographical location and fish consumption is relatively high vitamin D levels. It turns out that vitamin D, best known for its role in maintaining strong bones, is also needed to make new muscle and to regulate the immune system. Recent studies have determined that three of every four Americans do not get enough vitamin D, in large part because they do not spend enough time in the sun to make their own. The prevalence of deficiencies worldwide is comparable, especially in countries located far from the equator. Some experts have suggested supplements of 10,000 IU of vitamin D$_3$ daily as part of a regimen to control and possibly reverse MS. This amount is safe.

Dietary fats   In 1948, Roy L. Swank, M.D., proposed that a high-protein and high-fat diet was behind the growing incidence of MS. Until his death in 2008, he recommended that MS patients follow a diet that is very low in saturated fat. Swank was on the right track, but the problem was not so much large amounts of saturated fat as it was low levels of other types of dietary fats. Late in life, Swank recognized the value of omega-3 fish oil supplements because of their anti-inflammatory properties.

Myelin contains a substantial amount of fat, and, as with every other tissue in the body, the composition fat reflects what people consume in their diets. Changes in food processing in the twentieth century have led to the consumption of large amounts of poor-quality omega-6 fats (corn, soybean, and peanut oils) and trans fats (hydrogenated oils), which have pro-inflammatory effects, combined with a virtual elimination of omega-3 anti-inflammatory fats from the diet. Although increasing omega-3 fish oils won't likely boost energy levels, these essential fatty acids will reduce some of the energy-draining inflammation that is part of MS.

Vitamin B_{12}   Thanks to a chance finding by Edward H. Reynolds, M.D., of King's College Hospital, London, it is now clear that people with multiple sclerosis are almost always deficient in vitamin B_{12}. The deficiency often goes unnoticed if physicians look for signs of megaloblastic anemia, a sign of an extremely severe lack of vitamin B_{12} that precedes death. (Indeed, fatigue is one key symptom of vitamin B_{12} deficiency.) A better determinant of vitamin B_{12} status is to measure blood levels of methylmalonic acid.

Reynolds noted that vitamin B_{12} injections were given to MS patients as a placebo treatment, and he suggested reconsidering the vitamin as a real treatment. A team of Japanese doctors took the use of vitamin B_{12} a step further. They found that massive doses of injected vitamin B_{12} led to noticeable improvements in MS patients. The doctors gave the patients 60,000 mcg (60 mg) of the methylcobalamin form of vitamin B_{12} daily for six months. The recommended dietary consumption is a mere 0.4 to 2.4 mcg daily.

L-carnitine This vitamin-like nutrient (technically, a trimethylated amino acid) can also yield significant relief for MS patients. It is needed to transport fats into the mitochondria, where they are burned for energy. In a study of MS patients, doctors found that 3 grams daily of L-carnitine led to significant improvements, compared with the drug amantadine. Another study found that 2 grams daily of acetyl-L-carnitine also led to improvements.

Patients are often treated with immune-suppressing drugs to quell some of the symptoms of MS, but these drugs typically cause extreme fatigue. Doctors at the Pasteur Hospital in Nice, France, treated MS patients one of three immune-suppressing drugs: interferon beta, mitoxantrone, and cyclophosphamide. Because the patients had low levels of L-carnitine, the doctors supplemented them with 3 to 6 grams daily. Two-thirds of the patients had improved energy levels after three months.

Other dietary suggestions Gluten sensitivity (an abnormal reaction to proteins in wheat, rye, and barley) and dairy sensitivity might also exacerbate symptoms of MS. Although the link between these food sensitivities and MS symptoms is not consistent, it may be worthwhile to try eliminating all grain-containing foods for a couple of weeks, followed by the removal of all dairy-containing foods. If your symptoms diminish after you avoid one of these food families, continue to leave it out of your diet.

Matt Reverses His Diagnosis of Multiple Sclerosis

Matt was a typical teenager until he was eighteen years old and developed problems with balance, severe leg twitches, and an extreme sensitivity to temperature. A month later, doctors used magnetic resonance imaging (MRI) scans to document a dozen lesions in his brain and spinal column. Although he was an atypical patient (a young man), the diagnosis was clear: multiple sclerosis (MS). At that moment, Matt's future wasn't very bright. He saw himself in a wheelchair and began to feel depressed.

Matt's dad, Ashton, a scientist, read everything he could about MS. He realized that few researchers or physicians had seriously considered the roles of diet and alternative treatments in controlling MS. Yet such treatments appeared to hold far more promise than did drug treatments with their dangerous side effects.

Initially skeptical, Matt finally agreed to try the alternative therapies his dad suggested. One was a series of ten acupuncture treatments. Remarkably, many of Matt's symptoms cleared up. Then he began to eat a Paleolithic-style diet—mostly unprocessed foods, such as fruits, vegetables, fish, skinless chicken breasts, and a little rice. He also avoided all dairy, gluten, legumes, fried foods, and yeast. Finally, Matt began to take a variety of supplements, including vitamins, minerals, extra vitamin D, omega-3 fish oils, and gamma-linolenic acid (an anti-inflammatory plant oil).

A couple of years later, follow-up MRI scans showed no signs of lesions. Matt went to college, graduated, and began to work as a television producer. Despite the work pressures, Matt has continued to maintain his eating habits and take his supplements. Fifteen years later, he still has no signs of MS.

How to Survive Surgery, with or without Your Doctor's Help

Major surgery, such as for cancer or a heart-bypass graft, is essentially a medically induced coma, followed by a controlled semisterile knifing. Although surgeons are usually very skilled, the vast majority of patients do not receive adequate nutritional support, and, as a consequence, their recovery is handicapped. The food that is fed to patients in most hospitals is rarely fresh or nutritious, and the idea of simply ensuring basic nutritional requirements, plus a few supplements, seems alien to many doctors. As a result, patients suffer from postsurgical fatigue and pain far longer than necessary.

In a recent article in *Intensive Care Medicine*, Paul Lee, M.B.B.S., noted that vitamin D deficiency alone is likely to be a major contributor to illness and death in hospital intensive care units. The absurdity of the situation was shown in a study that found one-half of lymphoma patients to be deficient in vitamin D, but the deficiencies were intentionally left untreated.

If you are scheduled for major surgery, it is essential that you discuss any supplements you are taking with your surgeon and anesthesiologist. Both surgeons and anesthesiologists are often uncomfortable with supplements and typically ask patients to stop taking them for a week before surgery. Surgeons worry about excessive surgical bleeding and blood oozing from the surgical site, but neither issue is common. Anesthesia tends to reduce blood flow, and a small amount of oozing is not life threatening and can be addressed with a change of dressings.

Meanwhile, anesthesiologists are concerned about how supplements might interact with the chemicals they administer. (Part of the problem, anesthesiologists have explained to me, is that they have no idea how anesthesia actually works.) Doctors would probably do better worrying about the nutritional and biochemical impact of anesthesia compounds. Nitrous oxide (laughing gas) induces a vitamin B_{12} deficiency. Little is know about the nutritional impact of other anesthesia chemicals. So when discussing supplements with your doctors, consider compromising a little and stopping certain supplements (such as ginkgo, which is a potent blood thinner), but push back when it comes to vitamin C and B-complex vitamins. If you stop taking all of your supplements, this can increase the risk of surgical complications, such as infection, and slow healing.

In a study of trauma patients recovering from surgery, Avery B. Nathens, M.D., of Harborview Medical Center, Seattle, found that daily vitamin E (400 IU, given via a tube through the nose or the mouth) and vitamin C (1,000 mg, given intravenously) reduced the risk of pneumonia by one-fifth and multiple organ failure by more than half. Vitamin C might also lessen the risk of excessive bleeding, along with the need for transfusions. In the journal *Surgery*, Thomas H. Cogbill, M.D., of

Gunderson Lutheran Medical Center, La Crosse, Wisconsin, described twelve patients who suffered from excessive postsurgical bleeding. It turned out that they were deficient in vitamin C, and 250 to 1,000 mg daily quickly resolved the problem.

Aging increases the risk of developing a serious illness and the likelihood of using medications, both of which can result in fatigue. In the next chapter, I discuss how the aging process, the fifth circle of fatigue, contributes to a loss of energy.

chapter 5

Aging and Fatigue

Every living creature ages and dies, but the aging process does not occur at a uniform rate among all people or even in the same individual. Just as the Fatigue Syndrome and the first four circles of fatigue — lifestyle, eating habits, hormones, and illnesses — can accelerate or slow the aging process, the inevitability of the aging process increases pressure on the other circles of fatigue. For example, our ability to maintain an active lifestyle is affected by our inevitable loss of vigor as we get older. At the same time, aging often influences our eating habits — many seniors do not consume sufficient protein to maintain adequate muscle mass, and a lack of protein contributes to physical frailty. Hormone levels decrease with age, leading to more sluggish biochemical processes and sexuality. And age-related diseases and medications take their toll on our vitality as well.

We're all familiar with the visible signs of aging, such as wrinkles and sagging skin. As we get older, we also have less energy. Our bodies function less efficiently, and more is likely to go wrong. Little by little, we suffer the effects of "total system failure," although it is most often a failure of the cardiovascular system (such as a heart attack) or the immune system (such as cancer or an infection) that ultimately causes death.

Rather than be somber about the inevitable, it's important to recognize that you can slow down the aging process and take a big step toward maintaining good physical and mental energy levels. You can, of course, accomplish much of this by focusing on the first four circles of fatigue. In this chapter, I address many of the issues related strictly to the aging process itself.

It helps to distinguish the two basic ways your body ages. Most people think in terms of their chronological age, such as being forty or sixty-five years old. We all know, though, that some people look either young or old for their age, which is really more about biological age. Indeed, a 2009 article in the *British Medical Journal* noted that people who looked young for their age were in fact healthier and tended to live longer (assuming that their looks weren't the result of plastic surgery). You can assess your biological age, based on tests given at some medical clinics or a variety of free tests available on the Internet. These tests evaluate a variety of risk factors, including a family history of major diseases, eating habits, exercise level, and reflexes. They provide a rough gauge of your biological age, but with no guarantees for the future.

Why Do We Age?

In 1954, Denham Harman, M.D., Ph.D., conceived of, and began to expand on, the "free radical" theory of aging and disease. It wasn't until related discoveries occurred fifteen years later that Harman's idea began to gain scientific traction and acceptance. Although other theories have also sought to explain the cause of aging, most have revolved around cellular damage caused by free radicals.

Free radicals are molecules with unbalanced electrons. Normally, electrons come in pairs, but free radicals have either one electron too few or one too many. Unbalanced electrons seek another electron to reestablish a normal pair, and free radicals usually steal an electron from a normal pair, which damages part of a cell, such as a gene. Bruce N. Ames, Ph.D., one of the world's foremost cell biologists, has estimated that each of the body's seventy trillion cells suffers ten thousand free radical "hits" each day. That's an enormous amount of damage, and it eventually leads to a person's death.

Electrons play a crucial role in the movement of energy within the mitochondria of cells, and free radicals are produced as a normal by-product of our burning food for energy. Most of these free radicals are contained within chemical reactions, but a few do leak out. As we get older, greater numbers of free radicals are released by these chemical reactions and cause more significant cell damage. This type of cell damage is often called oxidation, and it is chemically similar to how rust forms on iron. According to Harman, our bodies' repair mechanisms fix most of the damage up to about age twenty-seven. After that time, the growing amount of free radical damage (oxidation) outpaces our ability to repair it. This cumulative damage is what we see and know as the aging process. In a very real sense, the energy produced in mitochondria gives us life, but it also contains the seeds of our eventual death.

As mitochondria become damaged from the free radicals they generate, they become less efficient in making energy. It's impossible to see the effect on a day-to-day basis, but it does become obvious after many years, such as between a twenty-year-old and a seventy-year-old person. Furthermore, these free radicals damage other parts of cells, such as DNA and membranes. Cell membranes function as permeable walls, allowing nutrients to enter and waste products to exit, but oxidation damages membranes and blocks these important transfers. Similarly, free radicals damage DNA, which interferes with the body's making of new normal cells and also increases the risk of creating abnormal cells, such as cancer.

To reduce the chances of free radical damage, or oxidation, Harman and many other physicians and researchers have recommended eating antioxidant-rich foods (vegetables and fruits) and taking antioxidant supplements, such as vitamins C and E. Antioxidants can squelch, or neutralize, many free radicals by donating an electron, which slows down cell damage and the overall aging process. Because of a recycling process that occurs among many antioxidants, vitamins C and E also replenish each other's missing electrons, enabling them to continue to curb oxidation. Although antioxidant supplements seem to go in and out of favor about every ten years, the totality of research indicates that they are safe, do slow the aging process, and do reduce the risk of disease.

Other Changes Occur as We Age

Aging is always the collective deterioration of our biological selves, but some changes seem to carry more weight than others. For example, free radical damage to mitochondria and DNA is particularly serious. Damage to telomeres, the tips of our chromosomes, which organize our genetic information, is also a grave problem. Each time our cells divide to make a new cell, telomeres get shorter, a change that eventually affects the integrity of our genetic information. When genetic information deteriorates, it increases our risk of developing cancer and other diseases.

Free radical damage is known to accelerate the shortening of telomeres, so antioxidants can likely provide some protection. One study determined that drinking several cups of green tea daily helps preserve long telomeres. In effect, seventy-year-old men who drank a lot of green tea had telomeres that were typical of sixty-five-year-old men. Green tea is rich in several types of antioxidants that do not occur in other foods or beverages, so this form of tea may have a unique protective effect on telomeres. Another study found that a lack of magnesium, which affects two of every three Americans, shortens telomeres and accelerates the aging process. In effect, two of every three people are aging faster than they need to because of magnesium deficiency.

Even if you maintain excellent eating habits and take antioxidant supplements, aging still takes a toll in many other ways. For example, aging reduces your ability to digest and metabolize food, so many people have vitamin and mineral deficiencies, even if they have wholesome diets. Part of the reason for this age-related change is a decrease in gastric acids and digestive enzymes along the entire gastrointestinal tract. One-third of people age sixty-five and older suffer from atrophic gastritis, a lack of stomach acidity that blocks the absorption of vitamin B_{12} and other nutrients. The situation is exacerbated by acid-blocking drugs, such as omeprazole, which interfere with the absorption of vitamins B_{12} and C and likely other nutrients. Inadequate vitamin B_{12} hinders the production of a wide range of biochemicals and can negatively affect neurotransmitters and red blood cells and result in gene damage. Most prescription drugs (especially oral contraceptives and antibiotics) impede the activity of vitamin B_{12} and other B-complex vitamins, and drug-induced nutritional deficiencies can also contribute to fatigue and the aging process.

You can reduce the rate of DNA damage not only with antioxidants but also with several B vitamins. Folic acid, B_6, B_{12}, and choline play essential roles in the synthesis of new DNA. Each time a cell divides, such as for normal growth and the healing of injuries, it must replicate all of its DNA—after all, DNA is the biological code that tells cells exactly what to do. Yet this replication of DNA is not entirely perfect. The genetic equivalent of typos creeps in, distorting those instructions for cells. Highly specialized enzymes scour DNA for these errors and correct many of them, but these enzymes also depend on B vitamins, such as B_3, B_{12}, and folic acid.

This DNA repair process becomes inefficient when people consume low levels of the B vitamins. The situation is especially dire when you consider that one of every four Americans does not take in adequate amounts of the B vitamins, and three of every four specifically do not get enough folic acid. Even with adequate B vitamins, however, the DNA repair process still falters (although not as quickly) with age. (For more information on nutrition and genes, please refer to my book *Feed Your Genes Right*.) Furthermore, the DNA that controls mitochondria does not benefit from repair enzymes, so this type of DNA damage simply goes uncorrected. These are additional reasons why our bodies don't work quite so well at seventy as they did when we were twenty years old, and they affect every aspect of our health, including our energy levels.

Folic acid plays yet another important role in regulating when genes "turn on" and "turn off." Folic acid is essential for making what biochemists call methyl groups, which consist of one carbon atom and three hydrogen atoms. Methyl groups attach to DNA and turn off genes when they're not needed. This ability to switch off genes is crucial in suppressing the activity of cancer-promoting genes. You want your body to do its very best when it attempts to turn off genes that can cause or promote the growth of cancer.

How to Slow the Aging Process

There are many ways to slow the aging process and improve your odds of achieving a long and healthy life. Some advice pertains to eating habits and supplements, which I discuss in more detail in subsequent chapters, and other techniques relate to lifestyle habits.

Restricting your calories   Certain researchers contend that the only proven method of extending life expectancy is through extreme and disciplined calorie restriction. Studies conducted from 1935 through the present day on numerous species, from rodents to primates (which are close biological relatives of people), have shown that reducing calorie intake by one-third starting early in life lengthens life expectancy by 30 percent. Similarly, cutting calorie intake by one-third in adulthood increases life expectancy by 10 percent. Furthermore, the animals on strict calorie-restricted diets have fewer health problems, including overweight, diabetes, heart disease, and cancer. In all of these studies, researchers have been careful to avoid putting the animals on a starvation diet; although the diets restrict protein, carbohydrates, and fats, the animals are provided with an adequate intake of vitamins and minerals.

Why would calorie restriction delay the aging process? Most scientists believe that consuming fewer calories slows the energy-production activities in mitochondria, and, as a consequence, fewer free radicals are created. With fewer free radicals, less oxidation and cell damage occur.

There are, of course, drawbacks to strict calorie-restricted diets in both animals and among the people who have voluntarily adopted such diets. The animals are hungry all of the time and don't let a crumb of food go to waste. People who follow a calorie-restricted diet tell me that their blood sugar and cholesterol levels decrease and that they feel much better, for the most part. Fatigue can sometimes be a problem, however, most likely because the very low intake of calories reduces energy production.

Cutting calories by 30 percent takes a lot of discipline, and the prospect of never eating a full plate of food simply is not appealing to most people. Yet I don't think we have to take such a rigid approach to eating to gain many of the benefits of a calorie-restricted diet. With three of every four Americans overweight or obese, cutting any amount of calories would prove beneficial to health. Just as calorie restriction increases life expectancy, consuming excess calories (particularly, sugary and starchy calories) shortens life expectancy. Given the large number of calories consumed by the average American—now estimated at 3,900 calories daily—cutting this amount by half would bring us in line with a normal level of food consumption. It's worthwhile bearing in mind that nearly all centenarians are either thin or of normal weight, not overweight.

Engaging in physical activity   A recent study found that a person's walking speed was closely related to his or her life expectancy. Walking was a general marker of health, and slow walkers were more likely to die, compared with fast walkers. Physical activity helps maintain muscle and good blood circulation, and it has also been linked to better moods and cognitive function.

Controlling stress   As I've already mentioned, the stress hormone cortisol ages the body and the brain. Therefore, it is essential that you find ways to manage the inevitable stresses of modern life. Some people can do this by emotionally detaching themselves and being less reactive to stress. For example, if someone yells at you, remind yourself that the outburst is probably symptomatic of the turmoil inside that person, not about you. This helps you defuse your stress. Other people use meditation, yoga, listening to music, and weekend activities to counteract stress.

Cultivating optimism, forgiveness, and gratitude Studies have shown that optimistic people tend to live longer than do people who are negative or pessimistic. There could be many reasons for this association between optimism and longevity. Negative people aren't fun to socialize with, so they may have a smaller social network— a risk factor for reduced life expectancy. Negativity and pessimism may be signs of depression, which could be indicative of poor eating habits and inadequate levels of B vitamins. Negative feelings could also increase the secretion of cortisol, the body's principal stress hormone, which damages the heart and the brain.

Instead of enjoying Thanksgiving once a year, it's helpful to practice it—in the form of gratitude—on a daily basis. No one gets anywhere in life without the contributions of parents, other family members, teachers, and friends. Gratitude is taking a moment to appreciate people who have meaning in your life. You can keep your thoughts of gratitude to yourself, or you can share them with specific people—and brighten their day. Meanwhile, forgiveness is about letting go, usually of resentment or anger. If you don't forgive other people, the odds are that you will do more damage to your own mental and physical health than to them (because your stress will generate higher cortisol levels). Reconciliation is a powerful human experience, reflecting a resolution of conflicts and forgiveness. Try it—the person you reconcile with may end up becoming your best friend and thinking the world of you.

Learning and engaging in creativity Slowing the aging process is not only about reducing your risk of developing heart disease or cancer. You also need to keep your mind flexible, adaptable, curious, and energized—in effect, on the younger side. New, nonstressful experiences stimulate the growth of new neurons (brain cells) and synapses (the connections between brain cells). In effect, the brain learns and adapts from these new experiences. The psychologist Ernest Rossi, Ph.D., has written about how specific types of activities can foster the growth of new brain cells and synapses. We should enrich our lives with humor, cultural rituals, spirituality, and being creative or enjoying creativity in others (for example, attending a music concert or a play or viewing artwork). Sometimes it can be a little uncomfortable to try something new, like going to an art museum for the first time. My advice is not to try to "understand" the meaning of a painting, but rather to simply enjoy the color and the brush strokes, in effect the illusion of using paint to create or exaggerate scenes.

In the next chapter, I discuss in detail how certain nutritional supplements can help protect you from many age-related changes and especially how they can naturally and safely enhance your energy and help you vanquish the Fatigue Syndrome.

Part Two

The No More Fatigue Energy Plan

chapter 6

Supplements to Jump-Start Your Energy

The nutritional supplements that I recommend can lead to improvements in all five circles of fatigue, thus helping you conquer the Fatigue Syndrome. They can help fortify your resistance to stress, strengthen the nutritional foundation of your biochemistry, enhance hormone production, reduce the risk of developing a serious disease, and slow the aging process.

Half of all Americans take some type of vitamin supplement, most commonly a low-dose once-a-day multivitamin formula. Yet high-dose supplements have a respectable following among millions of consumers and thousands of nutritionally oriented physicians. Over the years, vitamin supplements have stirred up a number of controversies, such as (1) whether most people should take vitamin (and mineral) supplements in general and (2) whether they need relatively large amounts of vitamin supplements. I'm convinced that most people can benefit from a high-potency vitamin supplement and several other supplements for overall health and to maintain high energy levels.

The controversies about vitamin supplements have their roots in the first few decades of the twentieth century, a time when severe vitamin-deficiency diseases, such as scurvy and pellagra, were common. At that time, most physicians believed that these deficiency diseases were the only signs of suboptimal intake of vitamins. In other words, if 50 mg of vitamin C daily stopped the gingival bleeding and reversed the fatigue of scurvy, doctors assumed that the patient was cured and was then getting adequate amounts of vitamin C. The problem, unrecognized by most physicians since the 1930s, is that scurvy and other severe deficiency diseases are not the first signs of vitamin deficiency but, rather, the most serious symptoms before a person's death.

Other controversies have stemmed from a clash of professional philosophies and opinions about nutrition. For example, many physicians and dietitians have argued that a person can get all of the vitamins he or she needs from following a balanced diet. Such broad generalizations have no scientific or medical basis, and there's ample evidence that the vast majority of Americans do not have anything that resembles a balanced diet. Only about one in ten people consume the recommended five or more servings of fruits and vegetables daily, so I could easily argue that nine out of ten people do not have balanced diets and could benefit from vitamin supplements.

Studies have found that most people believe their eating habits are far better than they really are. Yet even exemplary eating habits are no guarantee that the nutrients in foods will be properly digested, absorbed, and put to use. The only medically reliable way to determine whether a person's intake and absorption of vitamins or minerals are adequate is to measure blood levels of those nutrients. Unfortunately, relatively few physicians bother to measure their patients' nutrient levels, so their pronouncements of nutritional adequacy are unsubstantiated. One exception to this pattern is that measurements of vitamin D levels have recently become more common, which led to the finding that three-fourths of Americans lack adequate levels of this important nutrient. I believe that if doctors routinely measured blood levels of other vitamins and minerals, they would find numerous other deficiencies to be common.

Achieving Optimal Nutritional Status

There are sensible ways to approach the issue of nutrient intake. In 1939, Nobel Laureate Albert V. Szent-Györgyi, M.D. (who discovered vitamin C), suggested that doctors give serious thought to using optimal amounts of vitamin C, as opposed to the minimum requirements to prevent scurvy. He used the Latin phrase *dosis optima quotidiana*, meaning the quantity of vitamins that is needed to achieve optimal health. In 1968, another Nobel Laureate, Linus Pauling, Ph.D., published his concept of "orthomolecular" nutrition and medicine. Pauling defined *orthomolecular* as using natural substances to "straighten out" the molecules of the body. As an example, Pauling cited research showing that large amounts of vitamins C and B_3 could be used to optimize the biochemistry of the brain and improve health in general.

More recently, Bruce N. Ames, Ph.D., one of the world's foremost cell biologists, has also built a strong case in favor of optimal nutrition. Ames pointed out that many serious genetic diseases, as well as more subtle genetic weaknesses (which likely affect everyone, to one extent or another), can be offset by using vitamins to enhance the underlying biochemical pathways. It makes sense—after all, every pathway in biochemistry eventually leads back to its nutritional underpinnings. Ames also proposed a "triage theory" that explains how the body uses vitamins and minerals when intake is marginal or deficient. According to Ames, the body allocates low amounts of vitamins and minerals to the most crucial functions that are necessary to keep a person alive. The situation is a little like "robbing Peter to pay Paul," in that vitamins and minerals are diverted from roles that would reduce the person's long-term risk of developing heart disease, cancer, and other slow-to-develop diseases.

Ames has frequently pointed out that vitamin deficiencies are common and increase the long-term risk of incurring a serious illness. Indeed, at least three of every four Americans do not consume sufficient amounts of at least one vitamin or mineral. In my own conversations with Pauling, he suggested that people make a choice between consuming mediocre levels of nutrients to settle for mediocre health or getting

Percentage of Americans <u>Not</u> Meeting the Government's Recommended Daily Intake of Vitamins and Minerals

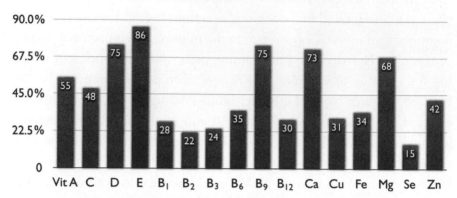

Based on USDA data at www.ars.usda.gov/Services/docs.htm?docid=10709 and Ginde, A. A. *Archives of Internal Medicine*, 2009; 169:626–632.

optimal amounts of nutrients to attain optimal health. The choice seems so obvious that I'm often dumbstruck that most people don't opt to be as healthy as possible. Sometimes, people are concerned about the risk of overdose from vitamin supplements, but this risk is extraordinarily small—in fact, inadequate vitamin intake is far more prevalent and dangerous. The latest data from the U.S. National Poison Data System show that not a single death could be attributed to either vitamin or mineral supplements in 2007.

I believe that nutritional supplements will play a key role in restoring your energy and helping you recover from the Fatigue Syndrome. They enhance normal biochemical activities (whereas drugs interfere with these processes), and I will explain in general terms how these nutrients work. None of the supplements that I recommend is a "stimulant."

Supplements That Boost Your Energy

In chapter 2, I explained the central importance of mitochondria in energy production and briefly discussed the crucial roles of coenzyme Q10 (CoQ10), L-carnitine, and other nutrients in mitochondria. In this section, I elaborate on these nutrients, discuss others, suggest dosages, and make product recommendations to enhance your energy levels.

B-Complex Vitamins

The B-complex family of vitamins plays diverse roles in our health, from helping us metabolize food to making and regulating our genes. Four of the vitamins—B_1, B_2, B_3, and pantothenic acid—are indispensable in breaking food down for energy. Much of the activity occurs in the "Krebs cycle," the biochemical process that burns glucose and fat for energy in the mitochondria.

Vitamin B_1 functions as the "throttle" that sets the Krebs cycle in motion. Pantothenic acid is necessary to make coenzyme A, one of the major chemical players in the Krebs cycle. At the heart of these biochemical reactions are nicotinamide adenine dinucleotide (NAD), which depends on vitamin B_3, and flavin adenine dinucleotide (FAD), which needs vitamin B_2. Both NAD and FAD help make ATP, the chemical form of energy in cells.

Vitamin B_1 deserves particular attention in this context, partly because high-carbohydrate (including high-sugar) diets increase feelings of fatigue. The breakdown of carbohydrates requires a family of enzymes called dehydrogenases in the Krebs cycle, and vitamin B_1 is required to make dehydrogenases. When people consume large amounts of carbohydrates, their need for vitamin B_1 increases. Yet refined carbohydrates (such as breads, pizza crusts, pasta, bagels, and muffins) do not provide vitamin B_1, so a functional deficiency of the vitamin develops. The solution is for people to eat fewer carbohydrate foods, increase their intake of vitamin B_1 supplements, or both.

B-complex recommendations: You'll find many good-quality and high-potency B-complex supplements on the market. As a general rule, I recommend looking for 20 mg to 50 mg of vitamins B_1, B_2, and B_3 by reading the fine print on the label. In most cases, the dosages of other B vitamins (which may be in mg or mcg) will fall in line. In terms of specific brands, I like the selection of B-complex or high-potency multivitamins (containing the B-complex) offered by Carlson Laboratories (carlsonlabs.com) and Solgar (solgar.com). Some people may need still higher levels of individual B vitamins because of stress or genetic requirements. In addition, some people may have high requirements for folic acid or vitamin B_{12} because of genetic issues. Elevated levels of homocysteine or methylmalonic acid are a clue that you may have greater needs for folic acid and vitamin B_{12}, respectively.

Vitamin C

When Mark Levine, M.D., of the National Institutes of Health, Bethesda, Maryland, was trying to determine the optimal blood concentration of vitamin C in healthy young men, he placed his subjects on a diet that lacked vitamin C. Levine expected his subjects to develop signs of scurvy, but after six months they did not. Instead, and to Levine's surprise, the first two signs of vitamin C deficiency were fatigue and irritability.

Vitamin C plays a multitude of roles in health, but two of them directly affect energy levels. First, vitamin C is needed to make adrenaline and other stimulating neurotransmitters. These are among the chemicals that keep the brain energized. Second, vitamin C is necessary for the body's synthesis of L-carnitine and related compounds, which are involved in the burning of fat in mitochondria. In one study, Carol Johnston, Ph.D., a professor of nutrition at Arizona State University, Mesa, found that taking vitamin C supplements led to a 15 percent increase in endurance among athletes, which was a sign of improved bioenergetics.

Vitamin C recommendations: Nearly all of the vitamin C on the market is ascorbic acid, the chemical name for vitamin C, although it may be mixed with rose hips, flavonoids, or other compounds. Buffered vitamin C may be easier on the tummies of some people, and you can purchase it from Allergy Research Group (allergyresearchgroup.com). Similarly, Ester-C is gentler on the stomach and may be better absorbed by some people. Solgar (solgar.com) is one of the few companies that markets Ester-C. Many companies sell packs of vitamin C powder that are supposed to be mixed in a glass of water, but most (if not all) of these products contain added sugar.

CoQ10

Discovered in 1957, CoQ10 is essential for the creation of energy in mitochondria. In the 1960s, the pharmaceutical giant Merck sold its manufacturing patents for CoQ10 to Japanese companies, apparently because Merck saw no financial value in them. Japanese physicians quickly recognized the potential of CoQ10, and it has since become the fifth most prescribed "drug" in Japan. A small number of American cardiologists began to study CoQ10 in the 1980s and have used it to treat patients. In 1992, however, the Texas Department of Health temporarily and inexplicably banned the sale of CoQ10—it was most likely the work of zealous but ignorant officials.

When I first heard of CoQ10 in the mid-1990s, I was skeptical of the claims being made for it. Could something really bring people back from the most serious types of heart failure? I learned that CoQ10 has one of the most remarkable pedigrees in nutritional biochemistry: it was the basis of the 1978 Nobel Prize in Chemistry. Without CoQ10, energy production would stall, and life would cease to exist. CoQ10's role in improving muscle energy levels has been demonstrated most clearly in studies of people with heart failure and muscular dystrophy. Because every cell contains mitochondria, however, and thus depends on CoQ10, supplements can benefit a wide range of health problems.

CoQ10 is often used to treat mitochondrial myopathies, genetic defects in energy production that result in extreme fatigue as a common symptom. Yet plenty of evidence indicates that CoQ10 can help people who simply feel fatigued. In a small study, Peter Langsjoen, M.D., of Tyler, Texas, asked several generally healthy octogenarian patients to take CoQ10 supplements. The average dosage was about 200 mg daily. All of the patients reported improved energy levels. One man gained enough energy to resume chopping wood, a pastime that advancing age had previously forced him to give up.

Recent studies have confirmed that CoQ10 supplements boost energy levels and enhance stamina. In one study, Japanese researchers reported that people were able to cycle faster and had quicker recovery times after only one week of taking 300 mg of CoQ10 daily. Another study, conducted at Baylor University in Waco, Texas, also found that both trained and untrained men and women had greater endurance after taking 200 mg of CoQ10 for two weeks.

CoQ10 has other benefits as well. A major study found that very large amounts of CoQ10 (1,200 mg daily) significantly slow the progression of Parkinson's disease, apparently by boosting the energy of brain cells. There's some tantalizing evidence that CoQ10 might reduce the risk of recurrent breast cancer and possibly other types of cancer as well. One small study found that it also slowed the progression of HIV infection. The researchers in these studies noted that CoQ10 did not seem to have any direct anticancer or antiviral properties. Rather, CoQ10 seemed to enhance the body's immune system, so that it could do a better job of fighting both cancer cells and HIV.

Some doctors believe that migraine headaches result in part from a lack of energy in certain brain cells. A Swiss study of forty-two patients found that taking 100 mg of CoQ10 three times daily led to significant improvements in about half of the patients. Two other nutrients, vitamin B_2 (400 mg daily) and magnesium (400 mg daily), have each shown beneficial results in reducing the occurrence and duration of migraine headaches. Both vitamin B_2 and magnesium play important roles in mitochondrial energy production.

Cholesterol-lowering statin drugs, such as Lipitor (atorvastin), are among the most widely prescribed medications in the world. These drugs block an enzyme that is involved in making cholesterol, but the same enzyme is needed to make CoQ10. Many of the side effects of statin drugs are related to CoQ10 depletion. CoQ10 supplements can usually prevent the side effects.

In the medical journal *Biofactors*, Langsjoen described fifty heart patients he had treated for adverse statin side effects, such as muscle pain, fatigue, difficulty in breathing, and nerve pain or numbness. He referred to the collective symptoms as "statin cardiomyopathy." Langs- joen asked the patients to stop taking their statin drugs and instead take

CoQ10 supplements, with an average dose of 240 mg daily. After almost two years of follow-up, Langsjoen reported a significant reduction in statin-related symptoms, as well as either stable or improved heart function. The number of patients complaining of fatigue decreased from 84 to 16 percent, and the prevalence of muscle pain among the patients declined from 64 to 6 percent.

CoQ10 recommendations: To reduce fatigue, I recommend 100 to 200 mg of CoQ10 daily. If you have CFS or are past age seventy, you can take 300 mg daily and more if your physician recommends a higher dose. You can use lower dosages, however, when combining CoQ10 with some of the other supplements I discuss in this section, particularly L-carnitine (or acetyl-L-carnitine), alpha-lipoic acid, ribose, creatine monohydrate, and quercetin. Physicians who treat cardiomyopathy or heart failure generally use dosages that range from 300 to 400 mg daily. This range may also reduce the risk of recurrent cancer. In one study, researchers found that 1,200 mg of CoQ10 significantly slowed the progression of Parkinson's disease.

Most of the CoQ10 supplements on the market are, chemically speaking, ubiquinone. A few of the supplements are a slightly different form, ubiquinol, which is more expensive but may be better absorbed by some people. In terms of specific brands, I recommend several products. Vitaline CoQ10 has been used successfully in a few major clinical trials, proving its effectiveness. These supplements also contain vitamin E and a small amount of sugar in a chewable wafer. They are sold by Enzymatic Therapy (www.enzymatictherapy.com/vitalineformulas/) and other companies. Carlson (carlsonlabs.com) and Solgar (solgar.com) also sell excellent CoQ10 supplements. Juvenon (juvenon.com) sells a supplement that contains both CoQ10 and acetyl-L-carnitine, a highly effective form of L-carnitine. Because CoQ10 is fat soluble, take these supplements with a little food to enhance their absorption. One of my favorite combination supplements, which contains CoQ10, L-carnitine, and alpha-lipoic acid, is Carlson's Nutra-Support Energy: Natural Fatigue Fighter supplement.

Jason Finds More Energy with CoQ10

Jason figured that he knew everything there was to know about energy — or the lack of it. After a long day at work, he would settle down on his sofa, watch television, and then fall asleep. That changed after he started to take CoQ10 supplements.

Jason was fifty years old, a time when many people talk about being tired much of the time. I find that many of my clients in this age group are suffering from the Fatigue Syndrome. Yet after taking 100 mg of CoQ10 daily, Jason felt as if he regained the energy levels that he'd had about fifteen years earlier. Now, he says, he has the energy to occasionally go out to dinner and a movie.

Yet Jason gained more than physical energy. Before taking CoQ10 supplements, he felt as if he agonized over the simplest decisions. New assignments and tasks at work were difficult to learn, and Jason was increasingly forgetful. The CoQ10 supplements sharpened Jason's mind. He says that his ability to learn and remember is now as good as it was when he was younger.

L-Carnitine and Acetyl-L-Carnitine

L-Carnitine and acetyl-L-carnitine are the two most common forms of the same vitamin-like substance. Various forms of carnitine help transport fat into biochemical activities in mitochondria, where the fat is burned for energy. L-carnitine and acetyl-L-carnitine enhance energy production, and they work with CoQ10 and other nutrients to support normal mitochondrial activities.

Earlier, I described the use of L-carnitine supplements to ease fatigue in people with multiple sclerosis. It has benefits for other types of fatigue as well. In a study of sixty-six centenarians, doctors found that taking 2 grams of L-carnitine daily led to significant improvements in physical and mental energy, along with beneficial results in cognition and muscle mass. Many drugs, including the antiseizure medication valproic acid, interfere with L-carnitine and, consequently, zap energy levels. Adding L-carnitine will not alter the effectiveness of these drugs, but it can protect against drug-related fatigue.

Animal studies conducted at the University of California and Oregon State University have found that a combination of acetyl-L-carnitine and alpha-lipoic acid (see the next section in this chapter) can boost both physical and mental energy levels. In the studies, old laboratory rats regained the abilities of young animals. According to the researchers, the effect was comparable to a seventy-five-year-old man gaining the vigor of someone half his age. A study of the effects of these two nutritional compounds on people showed that taking the supplements led to improvements, although they didn't transform seniors into middle-aged women.

L-carnitine and acetyl-L-carnitine recommendations: L-carnitine is widely available as a supplement, and, based on the research, it certainly seems to improve energy levels. Acetyl-L-carnitine is more expensive, but it does seem to be more biologically active, especially with respect to improving mental fuzziness. If you regularly feel tired, take 2,000 mg of L-carnitine with a high-protein, low-carbohydrate dinner; odds are, you'll wake up with more energy the next morning. Eat a high-protein breakfast (such as eggs and some berries, but no juice or toast) and take 2,000 mg more of L-carnitine. If this approach works for you, keep taking 1,000 to 2,000 mg of L-carnitine daily.

I like Solgar's Liquid L-Carnitine and 1,000 mg Acetyl-L-Carnitine tablets and Carlson's L-carnitine capsules. Both products are sold in health and natural food stores, and more information about them can be found on the Solgar (solgar.com) and Carlson (carlsonlabs.com) Web sites.

Betty Gets a Second Chance at Life with CoQ10 and L-Carnitine

By the time she celebrated her fiftieth birthday, Betty was feeling worse than she ever had before. She had trouble catching her breath and most of the time felt totally wiped out. She had to struggle just to walk from her bedroom to the bathroom.

Betty was diagnosed with cardiomyopathy, a catastrophic weakening of the heart muscle, and her doctor's prognosis was grim: she would probably be dead within a few years. Yet Betty had luck on her side. Three years later, in 1984, her cardiologist asked her to join the first U.S. study testing the effects of CoQ10. After taking 100 mg daily for four months, Betty felt noticeably better. Her heart was stronger, and her energy levels had improved.

A few years later, Betty increased her CoQ10 intake to 240 mg daily and also added 500 mg of L-carnitine. It was the right thing to do. Twenty years later, she was still active in her community and occasionally traveling. Betty lived for almost thirty years after her initial diagnosis—an almost unheard-of length of survival for someone with cardiomyopathy. On one occasion when I talked with her, she said, "As far as I'm concerned, CoQ10 has given me my life. I won't ever give it up."

Alpha-Lipoic Acid and R-Lipoic Acid

Alpha-lipoic acid, an antioxidant, has been sold as a prescription drug in Germany for more than fifty years. It has been used chiefly to treat diabetic nerve disease (polyneuropathy), improve glucose tolerance, and reverse *Amanita* mushroom poisoning. Although lipoic acid (as it is commonly known) has many cell-protective benefits, its principal function is to foster energy production in mitochondria. Indeed, many of its health benefits can be attributed to boosting the energy output of liver, brain, and nerve cells.

In a published case history, European doctors described how they used lipoic acid to increase levels of ATP in a woman who had extraordinarily low energy. As a child, the woman had been thin, weak, and exercise-intolerant. By her early twenties, she had developed eye-muscle disorders and droopy eyelids. On examination in her early thirties, she had very weak arm and leg muscles. Tests found that her body's cells were producing low levels of ATP. At age thirty-three, she was given 200 mg of alpha-lipoic acid three times daily. After several months, tests indicated that her ATP production had increased substantially, and her energy levels had improved as well.

As I noted earlier, researchers in the United States have used a combination of lipoic acid and acetyl-L-carnitine successfully to improve the energy levels of old laboratory rats and also, in a pilot study, of elderly people. To boost your energy, I think that combining lipoic acid with L-carnitine (or acetyl-L-carnitine) and CoQ10 is an ideal approach. The same combination of nutrients can also yield benefits with chronic fatigue syndrome.

Alpha-lipoic acid recommendations: The alpha-lipoic acid used in producing supplements is manufactured in Europe and China. The European product is usually of higher quality and more consistent, compared with the Chinese product, so ask companies direct questions about where they buy the raw material for their lipoic acid supplements. That said, even the highest-quality alpha-lipoic acid consists of 50 percent of the R isomer (the active form, which is found in nature) and 50 percent of the S-form (which is inactive). If you want to spend more money, you can buy the R-lipoic acid form, but, again, quality can vary significantly, so always buy it from a reputable company. Consider taking 100 to 200 mg daily of alpha-lipoic acid, and half that amount if you're planning to take R-lipoic acid.

Quercetin

Quercetin is an antioxidant flavonoid found in onions, apple skins, and many other foods. Supplements are sometimes useful in easing pollen allergies, but the most interesting recent research focuses on how quercetin increases the numbers of mitochondria in cells. The more mitochondria you have in your cells, the better your body will be able to metabolize glucose and fat for energy.

Most of the research on quercetin and mitochondria has been done by J. Mark Davis, Ph.D., and his team at the University of South Carolina in Columbus. Davis has shown that quercetin can increase the number of mitochondria in the brain and the muscles of laboratory rats. In both animal and human research, quercetin improves endurance. The effective dosage is 1,000 mg daily. In addition, quercetin may reduce the risk of getting the flu after strenuous exercise. I would certainly consider adding quercetin supplements to a regimen that includes CoQ10, L-carnitine, and lipoic acid. If you engage in more physical activity, this will further increase the number of muscle cells in your body, along with their mitochondria.

Quercetin recommendations: Cyclist Lance Armstrong and other athletes have been paid to endorse a specific line of quercetin drinks, powders, and chews called FRS Healthy Energy. I do *not* endorse these products because they contain fairly small amounts of quercetin (relative to the amounts that are needed to increase mitochondria) and far too many added sugars (including dextrose, corn syrup, sucrose, and fruit juices). If you want to take quercetin, skip the sugary forms and just get supplements from Carlson (carlsonlabs.com), Solgar (solgar.com), Solaray (solaray.com), or any of the other companies that sell them.

Ribose

Like many other energy-enhancing supplements, the benefits of ribose were originally recognized by bodybuilders who wanted to improve their recovery times, stamina, and strength. To make and recycle ATP, the chemical form of energy in cells, your body needs to use chemicals called adenine nucleotides, whose production depends on ribose. Ribose supplements can maximize the mitochondria's ability to make ATP in muscles, and ribose has been found helpful for people with heart failure. In a study of bodybuilders, taking 10 grams of ribose daily for several weeks led to increases in stamina and bench-press strength, compared with men who took placebos.

Ribose recommendations: To boost energy levels, I suggest taking 1,000 to 2,000 mg of ribose daily. Serious athletes may benefit from as much as 10 grams daily. As with other mitochondria-enhancing supplements, ribose works best if you combine it with a protein-rich diet and a little physical activity.

Creatine Monohydrate

Bodybuilders also pioneered the use of creatine supplements to increase strength, endurance, and muscle mass. Here's how creatine works: When

ATP molecules are used up, they get converted to adenosine diphosphate (ADP). Creatine helps the body recycle ADP back to ATP. Creatine supports athletes in their endeavors, and it can often give new life to the average person who needs a little more energy. Studies have found that in sufficient dosages (5 to 10 grams daily), it can benefit people who have muscular dystrophies, mitochondrial myopathies, and other disorders that reduce mitochondrial function.

Creatine recommendations: Start creatine supplementation at a "loading" dose of 10 grams daily for one week, to saturate tissues. After the first week, decrease the dosage to 5 grams daily. Beware of added sugars in powders or drink mixes that contain creatine. Many different companies sell creatine supplements.

I recommend a number of nutritional supplements that can help you fight fatigue and enhance your energy levels naturally and without any type of stimulant effect. These are my top choices.

Vitamin Supplement Brand and Product Recommendations

1. Carlson Nutra-Support Energy: Natural Fatigue Fighter contains a combination of nutrients that are involved in the cellular production of energy. These nutrients include CoQ10, L-carnitine, alpha-lipoic acid, and several B-complex vitamins.
2. Solgar Energy Modulators contains CoQ10, alpha-lipoic acid, and two types of ginseng extracts. Ginseng is considered an adaptogen, which helps bolster the body's defenses against stress.
3. Carlson Coenzyme Q10 supplements come in various potencies, including 100, 200, and 300 mg. Solgar CoQ10 supplements also come in high potencies.
4. Vitaline Coenzyme Q10 is the brand of CoQ10 that was used in many human studies with excellent results. It is formulated with vitamin E in a chewable wafer to enhance absorption. Other brands of CoQ10, such as those sold by Carlson and Solgar, are also good products.
5. Quercetin, an antioxidant found in onions and apple skins, has recently been found to increase stamina. Many companies sell

quercetin supplements, and I trust those from Carlson, Solgar, and Allergy Research Group.

6. Solgar L-Carnitine, a liquid supplement, provides 1,500 mg of this energy-enhancing supplement per tablespoon.

Supplements That Enhance Your Muscle

Energy is in large part about muscle—that is, having enough muscle tissue and mitochondria to burn food for energy, fuel your body and mind, and keep you ambulatory. Yet several common factors may prevent you from maintaining the muscle you need for health and optimal energy. First, you're not likely to make or maintain much muscle if you're sedentary. Second, if you're overweight, you have a poor ratio of muscle to body fat. Third, problems can get worse if you're overweight or diabetic because fat starts to accumulate around muscle fibers, further compromising your ability to burn food for energy. Fourth, as you age, you lose muscle tissue, so the older you are, the more of a concerted effort you'll have to make to maintain muscle or to slow its loss.

Proteins and Amino Acids

Proteins and related molecules called peptides are made from amino acids. Proteins have diverse roles in the body, and by some estimates, our bodies convert dietary protein and amino acids into two million different proteins. Not surprisingly, biochemists consider proteins to be the workhorses of the body.

Muscle is primarily protein (a steak is muscle from a cow), and the muscles supporting your legs, arms, and back are where you burn most of your food for energy. It becomes increasingly difficult, however, to maintain your muscle tissue as you age. If you are not physically active, you lose about 0.5 (one-half) percent of muscle each year between age twenty-five and sixty. During your sixties, you lose about 1 percent of your muscle each year—again, if you do not exercise. From age seventy on, your loss of muscle doubles with each decade. Doctors call the age-related loss of muscle protein *sarcopenia*.

Adequate protein consumption is crucial for maintaining your muscle and energy levels. Many people don't consume sufficient protein for several reasons. One is that they might have heard that high-protein diets are dangerous, and they consequently assumed that protein is dangerous as well—which is not true. Another reason is that ounce for ounce, good-quality protein generally costs more than starch (carbohydrate), so people on tight budgets might consume less protein. Still another reason is food cravings, which are usually for sugary or starchy foods, not for protein. And finally, many seniors simply don't have much of an appetite, which further reduces their protein intake.

I wrote about the importance of dietary protein earlier, and I'll come back to it in the next chapter. For now, I'll focus on how amino acid supplements can help you increase and maintain muscle. Many of the studies have been conducted on older adults, but the benefits can apply to any adult. These supplements won't magically give you a physique like a young Arnold Schwarzenegger's, but they can reverse age-related muscle loss.

Multi–amino acids   Scientists consider ten dietary amino acids essential because the body cannot make them. Another ten dietary amino acids have been deemed "nonessential" because the body can make them. Yet all of the dietary amino acids are needed for health, and some people have difficulty making the so-called nonessential amino acids. One of my favorite supplements is a blend that contains eight to eleven individual amino acids. In a study reported in the *American Journal of Cardiology*, daily multi–amino acid supplements led to significant increases in muscle after six months—and even more muscle after sixteen months.

Branched chain amino acids (BCAAs)   Widely used by bodybuilders, BCAAs form about one-third of the protein found in muscle, and they help convert protein into muscle. BCAAs consist of L-leucine, L-isoleucine, and L-valine. Sometimes all three amino acids are taken as supplements, and other times only L-leucine. Recently, Dutch researchers asked older men to take 3 grams of L-leucine, along with more dietary protein. The supplements quickly increased muscle synthesis in the older men, almost to the same level as in the young men.

L-ornithine Taking 2 grams of this amino acid daily for seven days, followed by 6,000 mg for one day, boosted energy levels and reduced fatigue in people who underwent tests on exercise bicycles, according to a study in *Nutrition Research*. Women seemed to benefit from L-ornithine a little more than men.

Beta-alanine A study of twenty-six middle-aged and elderly men and women found that beta-alanine supplements led to a 25 percent improvement in endurance and fatigue when they trained on exercise bicycles. The subjects were given either beta-alanine (800 mg) or placebos daily for three months.

Amino acid recommendations: Most amino acid supplements are produced from nonanimal sources, so they are compatible with vegetarian diets. I generally recommend multi–amino acid supplements, typically 5 to 10 grams once or twice daily. You can also opt for BCAA supplements, 3 to 5 grams daily. I prefer capsules over powdered drink mixes because the mixes often contain sugar. Also, amino acids might be combined with soy or whey protein—the whey protein is better than the soy.

Vitamin D

You need vitamin D for the normal synthesis of muscle tissue, and low vitamin D levels are now regarded as a cause of sarcopenia. In addition, a deficiency in vitamin D has been implicated in osteoporosis, falls, and bone fractures. Traditional thinking was that weak bones led to falls and fractures, but the current medical opinion is that weak muscles are the cause of falls and fractures. In this view, flaccid muscles, the result of inadequate vitamin D, fail to support the skeleton, setting the stage for falls.

Vitamin D recommendations: Vitamin D has so many health benefits, such as significantly reducing the risk of cancer, that it's simply dumb not to take it. Doctors at Harvard University and the Boston University Medical School have recommended a minimum of 1,000 IU daily for every infant, child, and adult. If you are dark-skinned, double that amount. Children older than age ten and adults will likely do better taking 5,000 IU daily. Opt for vitamin D_3, which is more biologically active than D_2. My favorite types of vitamin D_3 supplements—in capsules and drops—come from Carlson (carlsonlabs.com), but many other good supplement companies sell vitamin D_3. Do pay attention to the expiration dates on packages—vitamin D potency drops significantly after one year.

Antioxidant Supplements to Slow the Aging Process

Antioxidants protect against free radical damage, which ages cells and also stimulates inflammation, so antioxidants can be considered both antiaging and anti-inflammatory supplements. Antioxidant nutrients include some well-known substances, such as vitamins C and E and CoQ10, and many less well-known ones, such as N-acetylcysteine, selenium, lutein, Pycnogenol, carotenoids, and flavonoids. The richest food sources of antioxidants are vegetables, fruits, and herbs. You'll also find many antioxidant supplements at your natural food store and pharmacy.

Antioxidants work in many different ways. First, they are best known for neutralizing free radicals, the harmful molecules that cause oxidation. Free-radical oxidation is involved in every disease process, including heart disease, cancer, Alzheimer's, and arthritis. The scientific evidence strongly suggests that by fighting free radicals, antioxidants can reduce the risk of disease and slow the aging process.

Second, antioxidants have many nonantioxidant functions. For example, they play important roles in how cells talk with one another and do their jobs. When we don't have enough antioxidants, this type of cell-to-cell communication falters, and one consequence may be an increased risk of cancer. Third, many antioxidants serve as cofactors in chemical reactions. Vitamin C is required by a key enzyme to make collagen, one of the principal proteins in the body. Without vitamin C, you would not be able to make or maintain your skin, internal organs, or bones.

Fourth, some antioxidants have structural roles. For example, vitamin E is incorporated into cell membranes. In this capacity, vitamin E assists in maintaining a flexible cellular doorway, so that other nutrients can enter and waste products can be removed. Fifth, some antioxidants multitask—that is, they serve multiple roles. For example, coenzyme Q10 functions as an antioxidant, but it also assists in the production of energy. It helps transport energy-carrying electrons in cells, and this energy enables your heart to beat, brain to think, and leg muscles to walk.

Every disease process involves the free-radical oxidation of cells. Not surprisingly, then, antioxidants can benefit most health problems, such as those in the following list.

Health Problems That Antioxidants Can Help

Alzheimer's disease	Inflammation
Arthritis	Influenza
Benign prostate enlargement	Liver detoxification
Blood sugar (elevated)	Macular degeneration
Breast cancer	Memory problems
Cancer prevention	Migraine headaches
Cardiomyopathy	Night blindness
Cataracts	Overeating
Common cold	Pancreatic cancer
Coronary heart disease	Parkinson disease
Diabetes	Premature birth
Drug abuse	Prostate cancer
Fatigue	Stroke
Heart failure	Surgery (recovery from)
Hypertension	Vision problems

Antioxidant recommendations: Because there are so many antioxidant supplements on the market, I can't do justice to all of them and recommend as many as I would like to. Yet a number of products do stand out from the others. As far as individual products go, I highly rec-ommend Pycnogenol, a potent antioxidant complex derived from the bark of French maritime pine trees. It's sold by dozens of companies, but for general information on the product, start at pycnogenol.com. I also like the high-potency curcumin supplement called CuraMed, made by Terry Naturally. You can find more information at europharmausa.com. Both Pycnogenol and CuraMed are potent antioxidants and anti-inflam-matories. For combination formulas, I again recommend two products by Carlson: ACES and ACES Gold. The ACES product contains pro-vitamin A (that is, beta-carotene), vitamin C, vitamin E, and selenium. Meanwhile, ACES Gold contains these nutrients and ten others to pro-vide much broader antioxidant support.

In this chapter, I've discussed supplements that can naturally and safely jump-start and enhance your energy. A sound energy-boosting regimen, however, should be built on a solid dietary foundation. In the next chapter, I explain how eating habits can increase and sustain your energy levels.

chapter 7

Eating for Energy

During the last thirty or forty years, we have become increasingly removed from the appearance, texture, and taste of real, wholesome foods. The idea of a mother or another family member preparing meals from scratch is now considered quaint and old-fashioned, the consequence of social changes, stress, and a lack of time and energy to cook food.

Every day we depend on a variety of packaged and essentially prefabricated food products, from microwave meals to fast-food restaurants. All of these foods are highly processed—meals we ingest but that have little nutritional value.

As but one example, each day millions of people eat breaded and deep-fried chicken (breast meat, legs, and wings), shrimp, or fish. Most of the calories in these deep-fried foods come from poor-quality starch (breading) and oils (soybean, corn, or hydrogenated), not from high-quality protein—and definitely not from good-quality vegetables. A deep-fried piece of chicken bears little resemblance to chicken but has a near-universal look of a fat-soaked breaded nugget. These and other massive changes to the foods people routinely eat rob us of energy, rather than enhance it.

So, how can you change your lifestyle to gain more energy? In this chapter, I recommend ten "do and don't" Energy Tips to improve your eating habits and enhance your energy.

ENERGY TIP #1
Fresh Foods

Do Eat Mostly Fresh Foods

The number-one key to eating healthy foods is extraordinarily simple, but at first, it will take a little extra time and self-discipline to put it into practice. Eating fresh foods means avoiding nearly all foods that are sold in boxes, cans, jars, bottles, tubs, and bags. After eliminating these processed and packaged foods, you have plenty to choose from, such as seafood, chicken, turkey, lean meats, eggs, and most vegetables and fruits. You'll pick up the majority of these fresh foods at the meat or seafood counter or in the produce department of natural foods stores or supermarkets. There are some exceptions to my "no package" rule: olive oil, frozen vegetables, and frozen seafood (such as shrimp) are fine, as long as they do not contain any additives.

You may wonder how you will have the time and energy to cook foods from scratch. Let me reassure you: a 2009 study found that eating so-called convenience foods did not save any significant time, compared with chopping and cooking mainly fresh foods. My advice: you can save plenty of time by skipping the supermarket aisles that are filled with soft drinks, cereals, breads, cookies, and pastas. And once you begin to follow my eating plan, you'll notice that you have more energy to prepare meals.

Don't Eat Many Packaged Foods

Nearly every food that is sold in a box, a can, a jar, or a bottle has been processed and ends up having lower nutritional value than the original fresh version. As a general rule, packaging indicates that a food has been altered, most often with added sugars, salt, soybean oil, or trans fats. A little sugar or salt here and there may not seem like a lot, but it does add up quickly. For example, most of the salt that people consume is added to foods before they reach your table.

Nearly all canned vegetables have added salt, and almost every can of fruit has some type of sugar added. Another problem: Because of a loophole in food-labeling laws, companies can state that their foods contain zero trans fats, when they have up to one-half gram of these unhealthy oils per serving. Because most people eat more than a single serving, they end up getting a hefty dose of trans fats in foods such as crackers, tortillas, and other products. Breads sold in bags undergo substantial processing, and they have a very high ratio of starch to protein, regardless of whether they are white or whole-grain breads. Suggestion: Read the fine print on the ingredient list on any food packages you buy.

ENERGY TIP #2
Protein

Do Make Protein the Centerpiece of Your Meals

You don't have to follow a high-protein diet to gain the health benefits of protein. Protein stabilizes your blood sugar, which helps maintain steady, even energy levels. Some protein gets converted to muscle, the tissue that efficiently burns most of the food you eat. It's also easy to pick protein-rich foods that are low in saturated fat and cholesterol, if that's a concern. Suggestions: My top choices are fish, shrimp, scallops, chicken, turkey, eggs, and meats from grass-fed animals. If you like the taste of breaded chicken breasts, try preparing them with a light coating of Bhutanese Red Rice Flour (available from lotusfoods.com).

Don't Eat Low-Quality Protein

I consider most supermarket hamburger and corn-fed beef to be low-quality sources of protein. Meats from corn-fed animals have a high ratio of pro-inflammatory fats, which contribute to your feelings of fatigue and perpetuate the Fatigue Syndrome. Hamburger, in particular, tends to be high in fat and relatively low in good-quality protein. If you want to make hamburgers, I suggest using ground lamb, turkey, chicken, or a blend of these meats. In addition, soy is a very low-quality protein. Numerous meat-look-alike soy products use gluten to hold them together, which is problematic because many people are sensitive to gluten.

Protein Content of Food

Food	Serving	Protein Content
Beef round roast	3 oz	25 g protein
Black beans (boiled)	1 cup	15 g protein
Broccoli	1 cup	3 g protein
Brown rice (cooked)	1 cup	4 g protein
Chicken (white meat)	3.5 oz	31 g protein
Chickpeas (boiled)	1 cup	15 g protein
Halibut	3 oz	18 g protein
Skim milk	1 cup	8 g protein
Peanut butter	1 tbsp	4 g protein
Pork roast	3 oz	21 g protein
Shrimp	12 large	17 g protein
Tuna	3 oz	24 g protein
Turkey	3 oz	28 g protein

Source: University of California, Davis.

ENERGY TIP #3
Fiber

Do Surround Your Protein with High-Fiber Vegetables or Fruits

To nutritionally balance your protein intake, I recommend eating ample amounts of high-fiber (nonstarchy) vegetables and fruits. Roughly one-third of the food on your plate should be protein and the other two-thirds should consist of one or two different vegetables. (See Energy Tip #4 for my starch recommendations.) Nearly all vegetables are fine, such as salads (minus the croutons), broccoli, cauliflower, green beans, peas, spinach, and squash. You can steam some veggies and sauté others in olive oil.

Most people are comfortable eating fruit with breakfast and vegetables with lunch and dinner. My favorite high-fiber fruits are raspberries, blueberries, kiwi, and apples. The fiber in fruits and vegetables adds bulk and stabilizes your blood sugar, so they'll help you feel fuller. As a result, you will eat less overall. Fruits and vegetables are also rich in potassium, which can protect against muscle fatigue.

Don't Eat Potatoes

The common white and red-skinned varieties of potato contain a type of starch that affects blood sugar in much the way that an ice cream cone does. So if you have energy, weight, or blood sugar problems, avoid all types of potatoes. Sweet potatoes and yams have a little more nutritional value, but they are still very starchy.

ENERGY TIP #4
Starches and Sugars

Do Moderate Your Intake of Starches and Sugars

Two primary reasons why people feel tired is that they overeat foods that are made from processed sugars and starches, and as a result, they have either prediabetes or type 2 diabetes. Therefore, I recommend that people reduce or eliminate their intake of these sugars and starches (that is, the most common types of carbohydrates).

On a practical level, how can you judge the amount of sugars and starches that you can optimally consume? I usually suggest tailoring the amount to your weight, physical activity, and blood sugar level. If you're thin, you exercise regularly, and you have a normal blood sugar level, you can probably consume as many carbohydrates as you need for energy. Even if you can eat a lot of carbohydrates, I urge you to choose mostly whole-food carbohydrates, such as brown rice, yams, sweet potatoes, and fruits.

Don't Eat Refined Starches or Sugars

I am referring specifically to any food made with *added* sugars or starches, such as soft drinks, pastries, candies, breads, pastas, and bagels. The overconsumption of refined (or processed) starchy or sugary foods contributes to overweight, blood sugar problems, and up-and-down energy levels. They are called refined because they have had their fiber (chiefly, cellulose), vitamins, and minerals removed. Most processed sugars and starches are made from grains—think wheat and high-fructose corn syrup.

---

quick tip
How Your Acid-Alkaline Balance Affects Your Energy Levels

The concept of acid-alkaline, or pH, balance may sound quirky and faddish, but it has solid scientific and medical support. Kidney specialists understand the importance of avoiding acidosis and know that it's important to maintain a neutral or slightly alkaline body pH. It turns out that what you eat has a huge impact on your acid-alkaline balance, and this influences your energy levels and risk of developing many diseases.

The kidneys determine whether foods have an acidic or alkaline effect. If foods are acidic, the kidneys then send out signals to dissolve your bones to use their calcium and magnesium as buffering agents. Similarly, muscle tissue gets broken down to release ammonia. Conversely, if foods are alkaline, bones and muscles maintain their integrity.

Meats, fish, grains, and salt (sodium chloride) have an acidifying effect. All fresh fruits and vegetables have an alkalizing effect, and eating about 35 percent or more of your calories in the form of produce will keep your pH neutral. The alkalizing effect of produce comes from their high content of potassium and bicarbonate, even if the food tastes acidic (as tomatoes and citrus do).

ENERGY TIP #5
Oils

Do Use Healthy Oils

I recommend using several types of cooking oil: extra-virgin olive oil, macadamia nut oil, and avocado oil. Each of these oils has a similar fat profile and is high in antioxidant polyphenols and oleic acid, a good fat. Extra-virgin olive oil is sold at practically every grocery store in the world. Macadamia nut and avocado oils are more difficult to find and a little more expensive, but they have advantages. Both have slightly higher smoke points compared with extra-virgin olive oil, meaning you can use them to cook at higher temperatures. ("Lite" olive oil is processed, and you can use it at higher temperatures, but many of the beneficial nutrients have been removed.)

I find that macadamia nut oil and avocado oil can be used in certain dishes when you do not want the strong and distinctive flavor of olive oil. For example, I use these oils when cooking Indian curries. Macadamia nut oil has a subtle nutty flavor, and avocado oil has a slight, pleasant hotness to its taste. My favorite brands are Australian Mac Nut Oil (mac-nut-oil.com) and Olivado's several avocado oils (olivado.com). My top pick from Olivado is the company's rosemary-infused avocado oil — it is an excellent salad dressing when mixed with balsamic vinegar.

Don't Use Corn, Peanut, Safflower, Soybean, or Hydrogenated Oils

Processed foods usually use highly processed—and unhealthy—oils. The most common oils to avoid (or absolutely minimize) are corn, safflower, soybean, and hydrogenated oils. They contain large amounts of inflammation-promoting constituents that contribute to feelings of fatigue and the Fatigue Syndrome. If you refuse to buy the vast majority of packaged foods, you will likely avoid consuming these oils. Do be aware, though, that many commercial salad dressings use soybean oil (with added sugar or salt to make it palatable), and many restaurants (particularly Chinese) use soybean or peanut oil.

ENERGY TIP #6
Seasonings

Do Use Herbs and Spices to Season Your Foods

Herbs and spices are the most concentrated sources of antioxidant nutrients you can find. This is important because they help quell the pro-inflammatory and fatigue-inducing effects of stress and unhealthy foods. Yet more than being a great source of nutrients, culinary herbs and spices add a depth of flavor that cannot be achieved with salt and pepper alone. They tantalize the tongue and transform potentially boring dishes into stellar meals. Because of the flavor they add, herbs and spices can ease your transition to a healthier way of eating.

You can use many herbs and spices by themselves or try various combinations and blends. It's important to use relatively fresh herbs and spices—if they've been in your kitchen for more than a year, throw them away and buy new ones. I prefer the jars of herbs and spices from Spice Hunter and Frontier, but you can also purchase them in bottles or bulk from the Spice House (thespicehouse.com) or many natural foods stores. You can save plenty of money if you save and wash your old herb bottles, then refill them with herbs you've bought in bulk.

Suggestions: You can add oregano or a combination of oregano and basil (dried or fresh) to salads tossed with oil and vinegar. For a Mediterranean flavor, sprinkle the same combination on sautéed chicken. Basil and oregano also work well with garlic and lemon. Other good combinations include diced rosemary and garlic, rubbed sage and garlic, and curry powder blends. Another option is to buy premixed rubs for roasted chickens and turkeys, but check the ingredients to make sure they don't contain any undesirable ingredients, such as monosodium glutamate (MSG), sugar, gluten, or preservatives and chemicals whose names you cannot pronounce.

Don't Rely on Salt and Pepper

As a general rule, it's important to reduce your reliance on salt and pepper as your main spices. High-sodium diets are almost always low-potassium diets, and inadequate potassium is strongly associated with tired muscles, weakness, and the Fatigue Syndrome. You don't have to eliminate salt and pepper completely, but I do recommend that you cut down on your intake of them. Nearly all processed and packaged foods (even soft drinks) contain salt and sugar. The salt is almost always used commercially as a preservative and to enhance the flavor of an otherwise poor-tasting food; the salt essentially tricks the tongue and the brain into thinking the food is more flavorful than it really is.

Having said this, I do have some suggestions for using salt and pepper. First, I prefer Celtic Sea Salt and RealSalt brands, which are mined from ancient sea beds, undergo relatively little processing, and do contain trace amounts of many important dietary minerals. Second, I recommend that you use fresh peppercorns in a pepper grinder instead of preground pepper. Third, I suggest that you not add salt or pepper when cooking most foods, but instead sprinkle them at the table.

ENERGY TIP #7
Fluids

Do Drink Mostly Water and Teas

We are the only animal species that drink anything besides water. For a variety of reasons, such as our having a sweet tooth and being influenced by soft drink companies' powerful marketing, we now feel that many of our beverages must have some sort of candylike flavor. As I discussed in chapter 2, however, many of these beverages—particularly those with added caffeine and sugar—trigger frequent bouts of low energy.

Water is not boring. Its neutral taste allows the real flavor of your meal to tantalize your tongue. If you want to jazz up the flavor of your water, though, you can do so easily and inexpensively. (After all, soft drinks cost about the same as gasoline.) A squeeze of fresh lime, lemon, or orange provides a palate-cleansing flavor that allows you to enjoy the taste of your meal, in contrast to a caramel-flavored cola soft drink that drowns out the flavor of your food. You can use filtered tap water or bottled sparkling mineral water. Another option: Two brands of flavored waters, Hint (drinkhint.com) and Ayala (herbalwater.com) add the essence of fruits, vegetables, or spices without any of the calories.

You can make iced teas with a variety of unsweetened blends, such as Celestial Seasonings' Red Zinger. I am a big fan of iced green tea, and my favorite brand is sold by Miroku (miroku-usa.com); one tea bag makes a full pitcher. High-quality green tea, such as Miroku's, contains L-theanine, a nutrient that counteracts caffeine. Cheaper brands of green tea do not contain much L-theanine.

Don't Drink Soft Drinks or Energy Drinks, and Limit Your Coffee Intake

I've already explained how caffeine- and sugar-containing soft drinks, energy drinks, and coffee have bred dependencies and outright addictions. Yet one or two cups of weak-to-moderate coffee in the morning aren't a problem for most people. (Even small amounts of caffeine can be hard to handle for people who are hypersensitive to its effects.) Larger amounts of caffeine usually point to a serious dependence, and Starbucks is a particularly high-caffeine brew. If you brew coffee at home, I recommend using no more than one scoop of coffee per mug of coffee. A typical mug contains about 12 or 13 fluid ounces (just under 400 milliliters) of coffee, equivalent to 3 cups on a standard coffee maker.

Alcohol consumption is another cause of fatigue and mental fuzziness, and frequent hangovers are a sign of alcohol abuse. If you routinely drink alcohol with dinner and then feel tired the next morning, try giving up the alcohol for a week or two to see if your energy levels improve. If you have difficulty not drinking, you may be an alcoholic. I discussed some treatments for alcoholism in my book *The Food-Mood Solution*, such as nutrition, supplements, and joining a twelve-step program.

ENERGY TIP #8
Breakfast

Do Eat a Good Breakfast

What your mother told you is true: breakfast is the most important meal of the day. Consider the meaning of the word, that *breakfast* means "breaking the fast" of the previous eight or so hours. If you want steady energy levels at least through lunchtime, you've got to eat breakfast. But not all breakfasts are equal. A protein-centered breakfast stabilizes blood sugar, reduces your appetite for the next day and a half, and helps you control your weight. You don't have to eat a lot of protein, but you do have to eat the equivalent of an egg or a couple of ounces of meat.

Eggs are a great choice for breakfast, as long as they are not fried in an unhealthy oil. You can scramble them, make an omelet in a little olive oil, or poach them in hot water. I recommend having fresh high-fiber fruit as a side dish; frozen and defrosted blueberries are practically as good as fresh. You can also fold some pieces of leftover chicken or turkey into slices of cheese, and eat them with an apple.

If eggs and meats don't appeal to you for breakfast, another option is steel-cut oatmeal. A bowl of steel-cut oatmeal has a positive effect on blood sugar, similar to that of protein. You can cook up a batch of oatmeal over the weekend and then microwave breakfast-size portions during the week, adding cinnamon and berries for extra flavor.

Don't Skip Breakfast or Eat a High-Sugar, High-Carb Breakfast

Because many people think they lack time—often because they are too tired to get up early enough to make a real breakfast—they eat only cereal, toast, a doughnut, a bagel, a muffin, or an energy bar for breakfast. Or they'll just skip breakfast entirely. They are setting themselves up to feel tired within a couple of hours, eat too much later, gain weight, and drag themselves through much of the day.

A sugar- or starch-rich breakfast without any protein will turn your blood sugar levels into a roller coaster, leading to hunger jags and overeating and then making you feel tired enough to take a nap. Skipping breakfast is just as bad, forcing the body to rely on adrenaline, cortisol, and the release of sugar (glycogen) that is stored in the liver. These types of breakfast patterns, even in healthy people, result in prediabetes and elevated cholesterol and triglycerides, not to mention the Fatigue Syndrome.

ENERGY TIP #9
Meal Times

Do Eat at Regular Times

In addition to eating a protein-centered breakfast, it's also important to have your other meals at consistent times. I know this can be difficult with the pressures of many jobs, where deadlines can compel people to delay lunch or dinner or to skip meals entirely. Putting off a meal can lead to your experiencing a "blood sugar crash," characterized by tiredness, irritability, reduced concentration, and poor performance. Eating at regular intervals keeps your blood sugar relatively steady.

In practice, this means scheduling your main meals (breakfast, lunch, and dinner) about four to five hours apart. You may want to have a snack between meals, and for this, I recommend a slice of good-quality deli meat and cheese, an apple, or a salt-free homemade nut mix. (Put a portion of the nuts into a small plastic bag, and carry it with you in the car or keep it at work.)

Don't Set Yourself Up for Blood Sugar Crashes

When you delay or skip a meal, your blood sugar will drop and sometimes trigger the temporary release of stored sugar from the liver. Most people have a sense of when their blood sugar is crashing; they become irritable, weak, or headachy. The quickest fix—a sugary food or a fast-food meal—is the least healthy. It's better to keep some deli meats and cheese or mixed nuts in the refrigerator to help you get by.

ENERGY TIP #10
Portions

Do Eat Smaller Portions

When it comes to meal sizes, the general rule is this: the more you eat, the more likely you'll soon feel tired. The reason is that large amounts of food, not only high-sugar and high-starch foods, raise blood sugar levels; elevated blood sugar stops the production of brain chemicals that are needed for alertness.

There are other good reasons to eat smaller portions. Odds are that you are among the three out of four Americans who are overweight or obese, and smaller portion sizes can help you slim down and become more resistant to type 2 diabetes and heart disease.

Food and beverage sizes have tended to increase over the years. Fifty years ago, soft drinks were sold in 6-ounce bottles, not 12-ounce cans and 64-ounce bottles. Similarly, popcorn sizes at movie theaters have grown in size—today's small was once a large size. Many junk foods, such as pizzas, are heavily discounted with two-for-one offers, which encourages greater food consumption.

Don't Give In to Binge Eating

One change that occurred in food marketing during the last ten years is the practice of providing larger portions instead of lower prices. That was the idea behind McDonald's selling super-sizes of fries and soft drinks (which have the highest profit margin of any food on the restaurant's menus). At the supermarket or at big-box stores (for example, Costco and Sam's Club), package sizes have grown enormously. This type of food marketing makes it all too easy to eat too much food and to feel tired afterward. Even at home, the size of dinner plates has increased since the 1950s, so eating a full plate of food today means eating much more food than in the past.

Food binges and pig-outs are more than evidence of modern food marketing and gluttony. They are often indicative of food addictions, which have been carefully manipulated by food companies and restaurants to increase sales. Ironically, people are often allergic to the very foods they are addicted to, and the most common food allergens are wheat and dairy products.

How to Navigate Supermarkets

The typical supermarket sells an estimated thirty thousand food products, most of which you can ignore—and by doing so, achieve better health and optimize your energy levels. If you follow my first "do and don't," you can avoid wasting your time in the center aisles trying to decide which brand of energy-sapping soft drinks, cookies, cereals, and frozen pizzas to buy. Although it takes a little time to get used to skipping these aisles, you'll find that it's a liberating experience. You'll be in and out of the supermarket (or the natural foods market) quickly and with ample time to make a wholesome dinner.

The key to navigating a supermarket is to do most of your food shopping on the perimeter of the store, where you'll find produce, meat, seafood, and dairy products. (I explained this concept in greater detail in my earlier books *Syndrome X* and *Stop Prediabetes Now*.) You can buy some items at the deli counter, but again, you have to be careful to select less processed foods, such as real roast beef and turkey, instead of the type that is heavily processed and pressed (much the way that meats are prepared at Arby's).

The reason for shopping on the perimeter is very simple. This is where most supermarkets are electrically wired to refrigerate perishable (that is, fresh) foods, so that it's not necessary to run cables throughout the entire store. You can select your vegetables, fruits, meats, fowl, and seafood from the refrigerated cases. The dairy cases need a little more scrutiny because many products (such as yogurt and flavored half-and-half) may have added sugar.

How to Master Restaurant Menus

Eating in restaurants poses an additional set of challenges because you have little or no control over the ingredients that are used in a meal. Many restaurants buy large cans of food products, such as cooking oils, or they purchase already prepared foods, such as chicken and seafood, which simply need to be defrosted and heated. Although some chain and fast-food restaurants list the amounts of protein, carbohydrates, and fats in their menu items on their Web sites, they do not always reveal individual ingredients. In other words, Denny's, McDonald's, and other national chains of restaurants don't reveal that their ketchup contains high-fructose corn syrup or that their fried foods and desserts are made with trans fats. So the phrase *caveat emptor* ("let the buyer beware") is an even more serious warning in most restaurants than it is in the dietary minefield known as a supermarket.

When you eat out, you generally get what you pay for. A "dollar meal" will be just that—a small quantity of the cheapest-quality edibles for one dollar, which generally doesn't include fries or a beverage. When you add up the cost of two or three of the dollar meals, plus the side and a drink, you end up spending several dollars. You can do better, nutritionally, at the deli counter of a supermarket. So, the next time you think about getting a burger and fries, instead opt for about a quarter pound of sliced turkey, a quarter pound of cheese, an apple, and a bottle of water. Although the deli meats are far from a perfect meal, they are much better than a fast-food meal or prepackaged luncheon meats hanging from a hook.

McDonald's, Starbucks, and other fast-serve restaurants have nearly perfected the art of creating food addictions. Most of their foods or meals contain highly addictive and allergenic ingredients, usually in combination—for example, sugars, salt, wheat, dairy, and soy. Even a person with the best of intentions can have difficulty ordering only a salad when enveloped in the smell of hot french fries or brewed coffee. Arby's beef contains milk, wheat, soy, and trans fats. It's best to simply avoid these restaurants.

You'll do much better at many types of family-owned ethnic restaurants, but you must always read the menu carefully, avoid certain types of foods, and ask questions about others. (For more details about types of restaurants to choose, see my earlier book *Stop Prediabetes Now*.) I can't overstate the importance of asking questions about food preparation and ingredients, because descriptions on a menu may be very different from the concoction that ends up on your plate. I once ordered some delicious-sounding chicken at a casual but generally good Italian restaurant, only to watch the chicken breast and legs go into a deep fryer! So, ordering in restaurants is not the time to be shy and wimp out—your food decisions affect your energy levels and your overall health.

In general, your best bets are Italian, Greek, Japanese, Mediterranean, Middle Eastern, and Thai restaurants. Unfortunately, lunch menus are fraught with more risks than dinner menus, especially in Asian-style restaurants, because they have to sell low-priced and poor-quality lunches. Many Asian restaurants serve up essentially the same deep-fried and sugary choices, which you should avoid if you want to maintain your energy after lunch. Asian "rice bowl" restaurants serve mostly rice (an inexpensive starch) with a smattering of protein and a sweet sauce. Likewise, pasta is nothing more than predominantly starch. Eat these meals, and, odds are, you'll want to nap before you get back to work.

Greek, Italian, Mediterranean, and Middle Eastern restaurants tend to use olive oil, so they (and you) are off to a good start. Kabobs are pretty straightforward—meat broiled on a skewer—but they'll often be served with a cup or two of cooked rice, which is far too much starch for the typical sedentary person. Ask whether the cook can substitute a vegetable (other than a potato) for the rice. Avoid deep-fried entrées, such as falafel. In Italian restaurants, order meats or fish, not pasta, potatoes, or garlic bread, and if you're supposed to get a side of pasta, request a vegetable as a substitute. Most restaurants will try to accommodate their customers. A chicken Caesar salad, minus the croutons, is a good, well-balanced lunch, but ask whether the dressing is made with olive oil (as it should be) or soybean oil (to be avoided).

If you can afford to go upscale, you'll have a far better chance of eating healthy, fresh foods. (Sad to say, access to good-quality food is usually an economic issue.) Restaurants that serve fresh seafood, such as the McCormick and Schmick's national chain, are reliable and usually willing to modify meals for customers. So are many independent seafood restaurants and "nouveau American" and "fusion" restaurants that have inventive menus and often use local, as well as fresh, ingredients. Again, I cannot overstate the importance—even in the best restaurants—of asking questions about ingredients and preparation.

Lose Weight with Energy-Enhancing Foods

If you are overweight when you start to adopt my "do and don't" Energy Tips, you will likely start to lose weight. (If you're thin and physically active, you can certainly add more starch to your diet.) Although my diet is neither a high-protein nor a low-calorie diet, you will be eating mostly nutrient-dense foods. At the same time, you will avoid or eat fewer sugary or starchy foods that provide little nutritional value other than carbs and calories. Look at it this way: if you wanted ten bites of the most nutritious foods, you would opt for fish, chicken, and vegetables, not ice cream, soft drinks, or cookies.

The weight loss is a pleasant side benefit (as opposed to a side effect) of my dietary recommendations. Yet other factors encourage weight loss as well. Because your meals will focus on good-quality protein and high-fiber vegetables, your blood sugar will be steadier, and you'll have fewer hunger jags. Eating less almost always leads to weight loss.

Some people's biology is such that they store a large number of the calories they consume. Stabilization of blood sugar improves the efficiency of the hormone insulin, so that the body is less likely to store food as fat. Mitochondrial nutrients (coenzyme Q10, L-carnitine, and alpha-lipoic acid) may provide subtle benefits in burning off food, rather than storing it as fat. In addition, consuming more protein has a thermogenic (fat-burning) effect—it's slight, but it takes more calories to break down meat compared with carbohydrates.

In the next chapter, I'll give you food-preparation tips, offer recipes, and provide a meal plan to fight the Fatigue Syndrome and enhance your energy levels.

chapter 8

Energy-Enhancing Recipes and Menu Plans

It wasn't all that long ago when many family discussions and activities took place in the kitchen or the dining room. Food was more than simply love—it was the hub of family life. Today, breakfast is often ignored, and lunch and dinner are given short shrift. Sadly, both family life and food have lost their substance. Now, quick-to-prepare, hunger-quenching—but energy-zapping—convenience foods fill pantries and refrigerators.

To maintain strong and steady energy levels and overcome the Fatigue Syndrome, it's essential that you take the time to improve your eating habits. As I've already explained, you'll gain many side benefits, including a healthier weight and a lower long-term risk of developing various diseases. Yet one of the most immediate effects—often on day one—is more energy.

In this chapter, I nudge you to start to prepare and eat real foods, not the highly processed foodstuffs found in boxes, cans, bottles, jars, tubs, and bags. Good home-cooked food is more than just something you put into your mouth, however. The very act of food preparation — cutting, chopping, sautéing — is a tactile and sensuous experience, assuming that you have an appreciative family and don't feel rushed. In this chapter, I've tried to keep most of the recipes simple.

So, how can you deal with the hungry hordes (that is, other family members) while you prepare a meal? One way is to enlist their help, which means turning off the television, putting down the MP3 players, and not talking on the phone or texting. (Surely, you and your family can ignore these seductive technologies for an hour or so!) Another way is to have some appetizers on hand to pacify the ravenous tummies. You can serve a Moroccan appetizer consisting of a few unsalted almonds and a dried fig or two per person. You might be able to find some root-vegetable chips (such as taro root) at a natural foods store. Or you can offer a couple of dolmas, which are stuffed grape leaves in olive oil, available at many natural food and ethnic grocery stores. An occasional glass of wine among adults wouldn't hurt, either.

Breakfast

Breakfast really is the most important meal of the day. It might seem as if you can save time by skipping breakfast, but you'll pay the price later in the day with low energy levels and a bigger appetite. Many people skip breakfast because they are not hungry, which is a potential sign of abnormally elevated blood sugar levels. Having a bowl of cereal (which often contains added sugars), an energy bar, or a bagel or a muffin isn't any better than skipping breakfast.

When I began to do one-on-one nutrition coaching with clients, either in person or on the telephone, I was surprised by how quickly people responded to a healthy, protein-centered breakfast. Before consulting me, most of my clients had cereal, a breakfast or energy bar, or a smoothie for breakfast, and they felt totally out of energy by 10 a.m. After they tried my recommendations, my clients always called or e-mailed me to say how much energy they had on the first day of eating a protein-centered breakfast. If you're simply not hungry in the morning, you don't have to eat a lot, but an egg or its equivalent (such as two to three ounces or bites of chicken) will go a long way toward maintaining your energy levels through the morning. You can also eat a small amount of chicken, turkey, or meat that is left over from the night before.

SIMPLE SCRAMBLED EGG
(Serves 1)

1 teaspoon extra-virgin olive oil
1 egg

Heat the oil at medium heat in a small nonstick frying pan. Meanwhile, beat the egg in a bowl. After 1 to 2 minutes, pour the egg into the pan. Use a spatula to form the egg. Double the ingredients for a more substantial breakfast, and serve with some fresh fruit, such as a half banana.

SCRAMBLED EGGS WITH GROUND TURKEY
(Serves 1–2)

2 teaspoons extra-virgin olive oil
¼ cup ground turkey
½ teaspoon ground cumin
¼ teaspoon Celtic Salt or Real Salt
2 eggs

Heat the oil at medium heat in a small nonstick frying pan. After 1 to 2 minutes, break up the ground turkey (the equivalent of a small handful) into small pieces and sauté it. Add the cumin and salt. Beat the eggs in a bowl. When the turkey is cooked, drain off any excess fat, and pour the eggs into the pan. Use a spatula to form the eggs and turkey. Serve this with some fresh fruit, such as berries.

CHEESE OMELET WITH A HINT
OF ROSEMARY
(Serves 1–2)

2 teaspoons rosemary-infused avocado oil
2–3 eggs, beaten
1–2 slices of cheese, such as Danish Swiss

Heat the oil on medium heat in a small nonstick frying pan. After 1 to 2 minutes, add the *eggs*. When the eggs start to firm, carefully tilt the pan and use a spatula to lift the lower part of the omelet, allowing the eggs to run under the firmer part of the omelet. Do the same for the other side of the omelet. When the eggs start to gel, add the sliced cheese on one half, then use the spatula to fold over the omelet. If the eggs retain some of their gel-like quality, they will function like a thick sauce. The rosemary-infused avocado oil (olivado.com) adds a subtle flavor, but you can substitute olive oil. If the omelet is for two people, cut it in half with a spatula or a knife.

CHICKEN AND AVOCADO OMELET
(Serves 2)

2 teaspoons rosemary-infused avocado oil
3 eggs, beaten
½ avocado, sliced
¼ cup diced or chunked chicken, cooked

Heat the oil on medium heat in a small nonstick frying pan. After 1 to 2 minutes, add the eggs. When the eggs start to firm, carefully tilt the pan and use a spatula to lift the lower part of the omelet, allowing the eggs to run under the firmer part of the omelet. Do the same for the other side of the omelet. When the eggs start to gel, add the avocado and then the chicken to one half of the omelet, then use the spatula to fold over the other half. If the eggs retain some of their gel-like quality, they will function like a thick sauce. The rosemary-infused avocado oil (olivado.com) adds a subtle flavor, but you can substitute olive oil. If the omelet is for two people, cut it in half with a spatula or a knife.

EASY POACHED EGGS

(Serves 1)

Water
1 teaspoon white vinegar
2 eggs
Slice of whole-grain bread or 2 ends from a baguette

Bring 1 to 2 inches of water to a boil in a deep frying pan or skillet. Add the vinegar, which will keep the egg whites from spreading. Crack the eggs and slide them into the water. Poach them to the consistency you prefer, such as firm whites and soft or hard yolks, 3 to 5 minutes. Lift the eggs with a slotted spoon and serve them over a slice of whole-grain bread. Alternatively, create two cups by hollowing out the ends of a loaf of whole-wheat French bread or a baguette, lay the ends flat on a plate, and place a cooked egg in each end.

SCRAMBLED EGGS AND SAUTÉED VEGETABLES

(Serves 1–2)

2 tablespoons olive oil
½ to 1 cup sliced mushrooms
¼ cup diced scallions
¼ cup diced bell peppers (any color)
¼ cup cooked brown rice
2 eggs, beaten
1 tablespoon shredded (not grated) Romano cheese

Heat the oil on medium high in a medium-size to large nonstick frying pan. After 1 to 2 minutes, add the mushrooms and sauté for 1 minute, then add the scallions and bell peppers and sauté for another minute or so. Add the brown rice, then add the eggs, followed immediately by the cheese. Sauté everything together until the egg is cooked, 3 to 4 minutes.

Tips: Cut up the mushrooms, scallions, and bell peppers the night before. You can also increase the quantities of the eggs and vegetables, then transfer the leftovers to ramekins. Cover the ramekins, refrigerate, and microwave them for breakfast the next couple of mornings.

GERMAN-STYLE ANTIPASTO
(MEAT AND CHEESE) PLATE
(Serves 1)

2 slices roast beef
2 slices deli turkey or chicken
4 slices deli cheese, such as Swiss varieties
1 teaspoon Dijon mustard
4–6 cherry tomatoes

Arrange the ingredients on a plate. This is a variation of a common, casual German breakfast that's centered around protein but still a light meal. You can increase the quantities if you're serving more than 1 person. You can also prepare the plate the night before and refrigerate it.

DANISH-STYLE SMØRREBRØD
(Serves 1)

2 slices pumpernickel or other dark whole-grain bread
Choice of toppings

A smørrebrød (pronounced smur-er-brewth) is essentially an open-face sandwich. Two or three smørrebrøds are commonly served as breakfast in Denmark and other Scandinavian countries. The key is to use a very dark bread (such as pumpernickel). Spread some mayonnaise (such as Spectrum Naturals) or a little butter on the bread. Then add your choice of egg salad, chicken salad, pickled herring, liver paté, tomato, sautéed sliced mushrooms and baby spinach leaves, a roast beef slice with horseradish, or mozzarella cheese and pesto.

STEEL-CUT OATMEAL
(Serves 1–2)

4 cups water
1 cup McCann's or other brand of steel-cut oatmeal*
Blueberries or strawberries
Cinnamon powder

Steel-cut oatmeal has a stabilizing effect on blood sugar, similar to that of protein. (Rolled oats and instant oatmeal varieties do not have this benefit.) You can make 5 days' worth of breakfast oatmeal by starting its preparation in the evening. Follow the directions on the package for the amount of oatmeal you want to make. As a general rule, boil the water in a large saucepan, then add the oatmeal and cook for approximately 30 minutes. Divide up the oatmeal into 5 bowls or ramekins, then cover and refrigerate them. Heat each serving in the microwave for breakfast. Add blueberries or strawberry slices and cinnamon, to taste.

*Note: Some recipes call for soaking the oatmeal overnight before cooking.

FRUIT SALAD
(Serves 2)

¼ cup blueberries
¼ cup raspberries
1 kiwifruit, sliced
1 teaspoon cinnamon powder
¼ cup sliced banana
½ apple, diced

A fruit salad makes an excellent side dish to the protein portion of breakfast. You can prepare it the night before or in the morning if you have time. Mix together the ingredients. Add the banana and apple immediately before serving.

Lunch

If you eat a protein-centered breakfast, odds are that you won't be overly hungry by lunchtime. It is important that you eat, however, even if it is only a modest meal, to avoid a blood sugar and energy crash during the afternoon. Although some people still "brownbag" their lunches, the overall trend has been to eat in restaurants, particularly fast-food restaurants. It is difficult, if not nearly impossible, to order a healthy (that is, energy-sustaining) meal at fast-food and other types of chain restaurants.

When brown-bagging lunch, you have a basic choice between a cold lunch, such as a salad or a sandwich, and a hot lunch, which will usually mean reheating leftovers in a microwave oven. If you have no choice but to get a quick lunch in a restaurant, I recommend that you avoid fast-food restaurants and instead order a salad at a restaurant like Denny's or IHOP. Avoid all of the prepared salad dressings—they will contain soybean oil, salt, sugar, trans fats, or all of these undesirable ingredients. Ask for a simple olive oil and vinegar dressing (such as balsamic or red wine vinegar). Also, beware of the carb-heavy noodle salads at a salad bar.

SUPER-SAVVY LIGHT DELI LUNCH

(Serves 1)

¼ pound Swiss-style cheese, such as Danish or Norwegian Swiss
¼ pound deli chicken, turkey, or roast beef
drizzle of mustard, if desired
1 apple
1 bottle of water or sugar-free green tea

This isn't the most nutritious lunch, but it is far healthier than anything you can get in a fast-food restaurant. You can buy the ingredients at any supermarket or natural foods market, such as Natural Grocers by Vitamin Cottage, Trader Joe's, and Whole Foods. Lay a slice of cheese on a plate or a paper towel, place a slice of meat on it, drizzle on some mustard, and fold it over like a taco.

CEVICHE
(Serves 1–2)

This dish is native to South America, where each country seems to add its own distinctive touch. Basically, ceviche is marinated seafood that "cooks" in lime juice. Prepare it the night before, and take a lunch-size portion to work in a sealed plastic container or in an ice chest in your car. You can eat ceviche with a green salad, avocado slices, root vegetable chips (such as taro), or a few good-quality corn chips (from a health food market, not a conventional supermarket).

> 1 cup minimum of fresh lime juice, pulp removed (use at least 10 limes)
> ½ red onion, very finely sliced
> ½ cup very finely sliced bell pepper (red, orange, or yellow)
> 1 fresh jalapeño pepper, seeded and minced
> ½ teaspoon fresh black pepper
> 1 teaspoon salt, such as Celtic Sea Salt or RealSalt
> 1 pound firm white fish (tilapia, red snapper), bay scallops, or shrimp, cut into small pieces—or any combination of seafood
> ¼ to ½ cup fresh chopped cilantro leaves

Mix together all of the ingredients, except for the seafood and cilantro, in a glass (not metal) baking dish so that they are evenly distributed. Rinse the seafood, add it to the baking dish, and mix it with the other ingredients, ensuring that all of the seafood is covered by liquid. Add more lime juice, if needed. Refrigerate the ceviche for at least 2 to 3 hours before serving; 8 to 12 hours would be ideal.

CURRIED TURKEY SALAD
(Serves 4+)

This is a variation of one of my favorite and most flavorful dishes—I make a large batch, then eat it for several days and never get bored with it. Sometimes I'll have it with a green salad, other times with apple slices or spooned onto wheat-free crackers (such as Blue Diamond Nut Thins). I always seem to be tweaking the recipe a little. If you cook a turkey breast (see the recipe for Roast Turkey Breast with Rubbed Sage on page 180), this is a great way to use some of the leftovers.

> 2½ to 3 cups (1 to 1½ pounds) turkey white meat, cooked, cooled, and cut into chunks
> 1 cup diced celery
> ½ cup organic raisins
> ½ cup raw almond slices
> 1–2 teaspoons curry powder blend*
> ½ teaspoon ground turmeric
> ¼ teaspoon ground cayenne pepper*
> 2–3 teaspoons apple cider vinegar
> 1 cup high-quality olive-oil mayonnaise or canola mayonnaise (such as Spectrum Naturals)

Combine the dry ingredients first—turkey, celery, raisins, and almond slices—in a large bowl, and mix these ingredients together with a large spoon. Add the curry powder, turmeric, and cayenne pepper, and mix the ingredients together again. Now drizzle on the vinegar, and add the mayonnaise, starting with about ½ cup and adding more mayonnaise to suit your personal preference for creaminess. Allow the ingredients to integrate in the refrigerator for 1 to 2 hours before serving. You can substitute chunks of chicken instead of the turkey.

*Note: If you do not like or cannot tolerate hot spices, eliminate the cayenne pepper and substitute "Sweet Curry," available by mail order from www.thespicehouse .com, (847) 328–3711. (Although the Spice House calls this curry powder blend "sweet," it has no added sugars; it simply does not contain any cayenne pepper.)

LAMB BURGERS
(Serves 1–2)

> 1 pound ground lamb
> 1 teaspoon dried basil

1 teaspoon dried oregano

2 garlic cloves, diced

2 teaspoons ground cinnamon

¼ cup finely crumbled feta cheese

1 teaspoon olive oil

Lamb burgers are easy to make and reheat, and they have the rich flavor I remember finding in ground beef when I was younger. If you are concerned about the fat in ground lamb, simply drain it off if you're cooking in a skillet; if you're cooking on a grill, the fat will drip off. In a bowl, mix the lamb with the basil, oregano, garlic, cinnamon, and feta cheese. Form the meat into patties, thinner if you would like them well done and thicker if you would like them rare to medium. Heat a nonstick frying pan to medium-high and add the oil. Place the patties in the pan, and cook them for approximately 2 minutes per side. If you take the burgers to work, reheat them in a microwave oven, drizzle on some mustard, and enjoy a Simple Green Side Salad or a large serving of cooked vegetables to accompany the burgers.

LAMB MEATBALLS WITH SAUCE
(Serves 1–2)

1½ pounds ground lamb

1 teaspoon dried basil

1 teaspoon dried oregano

2 garlic cloves, minced

1 teaspoon ground cinnamon

3 tablespoons chopped cilantro

In a bowl, mix the lamb with the basil, oregano, garlic, cinnamon, and cilantro. Form the meat into meatballs that measure about 1½ inches in diameter. Place the meatballs in a glass oven dish. Preheat your oven to 375 degrees F, and place the dish on a rack in the middle of the oven. Bake the meatballs for approximately 15 minutes. Use tongs to transfer the meatballs to a serving dish or plates. If you take the meatballs to work, reheat them in a microwave oven, then dip each bite into a little sauce, and enjoy a Simple Green Side salad or a large serving of cooked vegetables with them.

> For the sauce
> Butter
> 1 shallot, minced
> 1 tablespoon apple cider vinegar
> 1 tablespoon dry vermouth or white wine
> ⅛ to ¼ cup whipping cream
> Salt
> Black pepper

Melt a large pat of butter in a small nonstick skillet. Add the shallot and sauté until it's soft (about 2 minutes). Add a little more butter, followed by the apple cider vinegar and dry vermouth. Stir. Allow the alcohol to burn off and the sauce to reduce. Add the whipping cream and stir. You can thin the sauce by adding more cream. Sprinkle on salt and black pepper.

Alternative sauces: Use some of the Italian-Style Tomato Sauce (see the recipe on page 192); you can thin the sauce with an equal amount of coconut milk.

Salad

SIMPLE GREEN SIDE SALAD
(Serves 1)

> Lettuce
> Cherry tomatoes
> Small cucumber
> ½ to 1 teaspoon dried oregano
> Homemade vinaigrette dressing

This is a simple and easy side salad that you can eat as an alternative to a cooked vegetable. Mix together the salad ingredients, except for the dressing. If you are taking the salad to work, keep the dressing in a separate container. When you're ready to eat lunch, add the dressing (see the next recipe), cover the salad, and shake the container to toss the salad. Tossing a salad enables you to use less dressing.

BASIC OIL AND VINEGAR
SALAD DRESSING
(Serves 1–2)

¼ cup extra-virgin olive oil
¼ cup balsamic vinegar
Other optional ingredients

Ounce for ounce, salad dressings are one of the most expensive—and unhealthiest—products sold in supermarkets. They're usually made with soybean oil, have too much salt or sugar, and sometimes contain trans fats and other undesirable ingredients. Mix the oil and vinegar in a 1- or 2-cup spouted measuring cup. If you plan to immediately use all of the dressing, consider adding one of several ingredients: ½ teaspoon each of basil and oregano; basil and oregano with 1 diced garlic clove; or ½ teaspoon Dijon mustard.

CILANTRO LIME SALAD DRESSING
(Serves 1–2)

½ cup packed cilantro leaves
½ cup extra-virgin olive oil
¼ cup fresh lime juice
2 teaspoons balsamic vinegar
1 small garlic clove, diced
Salt and pepper

Place all of the ingredients in a blender or a food processor. Puree until they're smooth. Drizzle the dressing onto a salad, and toss before serving.

SIMPLE TOMATO AND MOZZARELLA CHEESE SALAD

(Serves 1–2)

1 mozzarella cheese ball
1 medium-size tomato
Several small to medium-size fresh basil leaves

Slice the mozzarella cheese ball. Slice the tomato. Select an equal number of fresh basil leaves. On a plate, spread the mozzarella slices, add a basil leaf to each cheese slice, and place a tomato slice on top. Drizzle on extra-virgin olive oil, followed by balsamic vinegar. As an alternative, skip the fresh basil; after drizzling on the oil and vinegar, sprinkle the cheese and tomato with dried basil.

GREEN SALAD WITH GRILLED CHICKEN

(Serves 1–2)

2 to 4 loose cups (or simply eyeball a similar quantity) lettuce, such
    as Boston, leafy, baby romaine; or spinach; or arugula; or any
    combination
3–4 radicchio leaves, shredded
4–8 cherry tomatoes
1 small cucumber or equivalent, sliced
2 mushrooms, sliced
¼ cup sprouts or microgreens
¼ cup finely sliced red bell peppers
¼ cup finely sliced purple onion or scallions
½ cup diced cooked chicken
1–2 teaspoons dried oregano
2 tablespoons or so extra-virgin olive oil
2 tablespoons or so balsamic vinegar

In a large bowl, mix together the lettuce, radicchio, tomatoes, cucumber, mushrooms, sprouts, red bell peppers, onions, and chicken.

Sprinkle on the oregano. Toss. Drizzle on the oil, followed by the vinegar. Toss and serve the salad. If you are taking the salad to work, keep the dressing in a separate container until you're ready to eat lunch.

GREEK SALAD AND DRESSING
(Serves 3–4)

For the salad
7–10 ounces torn or sliced Bibb or romaine lettuce
15 slices English cucumber, each about the thickness of 2 quarters
10–15 cherry tomatoes
10–15 pitted Kalamata olives
4 very thin slices red onion
6 very thin slices red bell pepper
Optional: ½ cup crumbled feta or goat cheese
2 teaspoons dried Greek oregano
1 teaspoon dried basil

For the dressing
4 tablespoons (approximately) extra-virgin olive oil
3 tablespoons (approximately) balsamic or red wine vinegar
1 tablespoon fresh-squeezed lemon juice

Combine all of the salad ingredients, except for the oregano and basil, in a large salad bowl and then toss. Sprinkle on the oregano and basil, and toss once more. Pour the oil over the salad, followed by the vinegar and lemon juice. Toss and serve.

Options: You can adjust the amounts of any ingredient to suit your tastes. In addition, tossing a salad with dressing generally uses less dressing (and therefore has fewer calories), compared with pouring a dressing directly onto the plate.

Dinner

ROASTED WHOLE CHICKEN

(Serves 3–4)

You will need a roasting pan with a removable wire rack to properly roast a chicken. The chicken will rest on the rack, and the pan will catch the drippings that you will use for a sauce.

- 4- to 5-pound whole chicken
- 1 tablespoon chopped rosemary
- 4 garlic cloves, diced
- 1 to 2 cups high-quality chicken broth (for example, Pacific brand)

If your budget allows, use an organic free-range chicken—it will have an exceptional taste and be less fatty than other varieties of whole chickens. Preheat your oven to 425 degrees F. Take the chicken out of its plastic wrapping, and remove the giblets, which will be wrapped in paper inside the cavity. Rinse the chicken inside and out under cold running water, then dry the outside with paper towels. Use your fingers to gently separate part of the skin over the breast, and do the same on the other side of the chicken to create pockets. Rub some of the rosemary and garlic under the skin. If you have extra spices, insert them into the bird's inner cavity.

Roast the chicken for about 1 hour, and use an instant-read thermometer to check that the meat in the thickest part of the breast is 160 to 165 degrees F. If it isn't that hot yet, continue to cook the chicken for a few more minutes. A larger chicken will need about 10 minutes of additional cooking time per pound of weight. When it's cooked, transfer the chicken to a serving plate, cover it with aluminum foil, and allow it to rest for 10 minutes to redistribute its juices. The chicken will continue to cook for a few minutes while it rests.

You can use some of the giblets to make the gravy, boil them separately in water as a treat for your cat or dog (minus the neck, which has too many bones), or dispose of them. If you choose to use them, select the heart and liver and dice them. While the chicken is resting, remove the wire rack from the roasting pan and place the pan on one or two burners on the stovetop. Add the chicken broth. Use a wooden spatula to break up the drippings, but discard any that are very hard. Add the giblets, sauté, and allow the gravy to reduce and thicken, about 5 to 10 minutes.

Slice and serve the chicken, and drizzle the gravy over the slices. When the chicken cools a little, cut or tear off much of the remaining meat for subsequent meals. Save the carcass to make Chicken Rice Soup (see the recipe on page 194).

Options: As an alternative to rosemary and garlic, you can try these spice combinations: rubbed sage and garlic, cayenne pepper and paprika, tandoori spice mix, or poultry seasoning.

ROTISSERIE CHICKEN ON THE RUN
(Serves 2)

1 rotisserie chicken from the supermarket
Vegetables for steaming, such as broccoli or cauliflower crowns
1 cup good-quality chicken broth, such as Pacific brand
Salt

If you simply don't have the time to make a roast chicken, you can improvise with a cooked supermarket rotisserie chicken. It's important to avoid chickens that have any sweet-and-sour flavors because they will contain added sugars. The simpler the preparation, the better—with herbs for flavoring being ideal. When you get home, steam some vegetables, such as broccoli or cauliflower, which will take 8 to 10 minutes. Pour about 1 cup of chicken broth into a saucepan and heat it on medium. If you have any juicy runoff from the chicken at the bottom of the pan, add this to the broth. Add a little salt, if you wish. Meanwhile, tear or slice off some of the chicken, arrange it on a plate, and pour a little of the broth over it as a gravy.

quick tip
Spice Combinations That Work

You can add oregano or a combination of oregano and basil (dried or fresh) to salads tossed with oil and vinegar. For a Mediterranean flavor, sprinkle the same combination over sautéed chicken. Basil and oregano also work well with garlic and lemon. Other good combinations include minced rosemary and garlic, rubbed sage and garlic, and curry powder blends. Another option consists of premixed rubs for roasted chickens and turkeys, but check the ingredients to make sure they don't contain any undesirable ingredients.

ROAST TURKEY BREAST
WITH RUBBED SAGE

(Serves 4+)

Turkey breast on bone, approximately 6 pounds
Olive oil
2 tablespoons rubbed sage
1 to 2 cups chicken or vegetable broth

It's easy to cook a turkey breast, and you'll likely have plenty of leftovers for a variety of quick meals, such as turkey sandwiches and turkey tacos. Rinse the breast and pat it dry. Drizzle a little oil to coat all sides of the breast. Sprinkle sage on the breast. Place it breast-side up on the wire rack of a roasting pan. Roast it in an oven preheated to 375 degrees F. Set the timer to 1 hour, and use an instant-read thermometer to check the temperature. If the internal temperature is less than 160 degrees F, roast it for at least another 10 to 20 minutes. Transfer the cooked breast to a large plate or dish, cover it with aluminum foil, and allow it to rest for 10 minutes. Meanwhile, remove the wire rack from the roasting pan, and place the pan so that it straddles two burners on the stove top. Add 1 to 2 cups of chicken or vegetable broth. Use a wooden spatula to stir the broth and mix in some of the drippings to make a quick gravy. Spoon the gravy over the turkey slices. Leftover gravy can be refrigerated and reused for a week.

Options: You can adapt this recipe to a half-breast on the bone or to a boneless breast.

TURKEY TACOS
(Serves 4)

Olive oil
1 cup diced white or cremini mushrooms
2 shallot bulbs, diced
1–2 cloves garlic, minced
1 cup chopped spinach leaves, packed tightly
1½ cups chopped, diced, or shredded cooked turkey
½ cup crème fraiche
3 tablespoons snipped or diced chives
½ cup grated Romano or other cheese
4 whole-wheat, low-carb tortillas or 4 folded blue-corn taco shells

This is a great way to use some of your leftover baked turkey breast. Start by heating 1 tablespoon of oil in a large nonstick skillet. Add the mushrooms, shallots, and garlic, and sauté for a minute or two. Add the spinach and sauté until it's wilted. Remove the skillet from the heat. Add the turkey, crème fraiche, chives, and cheese, and mix together all of the ingredients. Spread the ingredients in a line in the center of a soft taco shell, roll it up, and serve.

TANDOORI CHICKEN TACOS
(Serves 4)

1 pat butter
1 tablespoon macadamia nut oil (alternative: "lite" olive oil)
½ sweet onion, diced
2 cloves garlic, diced
2 tablespoons grated ginger
1–2 tablespoons tandoori spice blend

---

quick tip
Healthy Pasta Substitutes

Too much pasta might make your tummy feel full, but it's likely to leave you more tired. Yet I do recommend two types of tasty pasta that, in moderate amounts, are healthy. Eden Foods' Buckwheat Soba is made in Japan from 100 percent buckwheat, which is made from an herb, not a grain. (Most buckwheat soba noodles are 75 percent whole wheat, not buckwheat.) Cook buckwheat pasta for 6 to 8 minutes in boiling water—do not overcook it. Eden Foods also sells Kuzu Pasta, which is made from a gluten-free plant root, also grown and harvested in Japan. You can find information on both products at www.edenfoods.com.

---

1 pound boneless, skinless chicken breast, cut into chunks
½ cup low-fat, sugar-free yogurt (Fage and Oikos are good brands)
4 whole-wheat, low-carb tortillas or 4 folded blue-corn taco shells

Heat a nonstick skillet on medium high, add the butter and oil, then sauté the onion, garlic, and ginger. Add the chicken and sauté, sprinkling on the tandoori spice blend. When the chicken is cooked, reduce the temperature to medium heat and add the yogurt. Mix the ingredients and serve them in either the tortillas or the taco shells. This recipe was adapted from one by Bal Arneson.

CHICKEN AND BROCCOLI STIR-FRY

(Serves 2+)

1 tablespoon macadamia nut oil or other neutral-flavored oil
2 garlic cloves, diced
1 tablespoon peeled and shredded or minced ginger
1 shallot bulb, diced
1 pound boneless, skinless chicken breast, cut into 2-inch strips
3 tablespoons tamari
1 teaspoon apple cider vinegar

½ cup good-quality chicken broth (such as Pacific brand)
¼ to ½ teaspoon red pepper flakes (optional)
1 cup small broccoli florets
2 ounces Kuzu noodles (optional)*

Heat the oil in a wok on medium high. Add the garlic, ginger, and shallot, and sauté until they're soft (1 to 2 minutes). Add the chicken and sauté until it's about half cooked (the outside of the chicken will be white). Add the tamari and vinegar. Add the chicken broth and red pepper flakes. Add the broccoli and continue to sauté for 3 to 4 more minutes. (The broccoli should be lightly cooked so that it retains some crispness.)

*Note: For the optional Kuzu noodles, cook them as directed—boil them in water in a separate saucepan for 10 minutes.

BUCKWHEAT NOODLE PASTA
WITH RICH RED SAUCE
(Serves 4)

2 cups tomato sauce
1 cup coconut milk (not lite)
1 pound ground turkey
Buckwheat soba noodles, 1 ounce per person
Romano cheese

Buckwheat is not a grain or a grass, yet it can sometimes be used like wheat. It is particularly rich in rutin, an antioxidant found in citrus fruits. It does not contain any gluten; however, some people are allergic to buckwheat and can have potentially severe reactions to it.

To make the sauce, bring the tomato sauce to a boil, then add the coconut milk and reduce the heat to medium. (See my Italian-Style Tomato Sauce recipe on page 192, or simply buy a jar of good-quality sauce at a natural foods store.) Meanwhile, sauté the ground turkey, drain off the fat, and add it to the tomato sauce. Reduce the heat to a simmer.

---

quick tip
Jazz Up That Mayo and Call It Aioli

An aioli is technically a mayonnaise flavored with garlic. You can use any number of ingredients, however, to magically change the flavor of mayo. Use the aioli as a sandwich spread, as a sauce of sorts when rolling foods in whole-wheat tortillas, or as a dipping sauce for baked chicken or turkey. I like to start with Spectrum Naturals Canola or Olive Oil Mayonnaise, both of which are sold at most natural food stores. You can add a little pesto, minced roasted red bell peppers, paprika, minced chives, Dijon mustard, wasabi and tamari (or soy sauce), chipotle powder, or curry powder.

Follow the cooking directions on a package of buckwheat soba noodles. The noodles will cook in 6 to 8 minutes; be careful not to overcook them. Serve the pasta with the sauce on top. Add Romano cheese, if desired.

SEA SCALLOPS IN BUTTER
AND WINE SAUCE

(Serves 2)

10 plump sea scallops (about 1 pound)
½ teaspoon Celtic Sea Salt, Real Salt, or generic sea salt
¼ to ½ teaspoon fresh ground black pepper
¼ cup Lotus Foods Bhutanese Red Rice Flour
½ stick unsalted butter
1 large shallot, diced
4 cloves garlic, diced
Juice of 1 lemon
¼ cup dry vermouth
2 tablespoons chopped flat-leaf parsley

Rinse and pat dry the scallops. Sprinkle the salt and fresh ground pepper on the scallops, then roll them in the red rice flour. Heat a large skillet, and melt about half of the butter. Sauté the diced shallot and garlic, then add the scallops. With a spatula, mix the shallot and garlic with the scallops, and turn the scallops over from time to time to cook them evenly, no more than 10 minutes' total cooking time. The diced shallot and garlic will turn brown and crunchy, adding a nice texture to the sauce. Add the juice from half of the lemon. Drizzle the vermouth toward the edge of the skillet, and tip the skillet to move it around. Add the remaining lemon juice. Finally, sprinkle on the parsley and serve.

TANDOORI SHRIMP
(Serves 2)

½ pound (or about 1 cup) sugar-free yogurt
Tandoori spice mix
1 pound shelled and deveined large shrimp (20 count)

In a large glass or plastic bowl, mix together the yogurt and tandoori spices. Add the shrimp, and marinate them for at least 1 hour. Place the shrimp on skewers. (If you use wooden skewers, soak them in water for 1 hour before using them to prevent burning.) Place the skewers on a grill or a wire rack of a broiling pan, so that the pan will catch the drippings. (Pre-coat the wires with a little olive oil to prevent the shrimp from sticking.) Grill or broil the shrimp for 3 to 5 minutes, turn them over, and grill or broil them for another 3 minutes. Be careful not to overcook the shrimp.

Optional: Brush melted butter onto the shrimp once or twice while they're cooking.

---

quick tip
Ginger-Lemon Iced Tea

Ginger is healthy and has documented anti-inflammatory benefits. You can prepare this as either an iced or a hot tea. Use a vegetable peeler to remove the skin, then grate 1 teaspoon of fresh ginger. Add the ginger to a glass of cold water, and squeeze in the juice from ½ lemon.

MARINATED CHICKEN BREASTS

(Serves 2)

⅓ cup olive oil
Juice of 1 fresh lemon
2–3 garlic cloves, diced
2 teaspoons chopped fresh oregano, or 1 teaspoon dried oregano, or
　　1 teaspoon chopped fresh rosemary leaves
1 pound boneless, skinless chicken breast, cut into strips or small
　　pieces

Mix together the oil, lemon juice, garlic, and herbs in either a large
bowl or a plastic bag. Add the chicken, and marinate everything for 1 to
24 hours. If you cannot completely coat the chicken with the marinade,
add a little more oil. Remove the chicken from the marinade, and sauté
it in a nonstick skillet until it's cooked. When sautéing, you can use
some of the leftover marinade instead of additional olive oil.

KOFTA KABOBS

(Serves 3–4)

1 pound ground lamb or extra-lean ground beef, or a mix of both
½ cup minced red onion
2–5 cloves garlic, minced
½ cup fresh chopped cilantro or flat-leaf parsley
¼ teaspoon ground cinnamon
½ teaspoon ground allspice
⅛ teaspoon ground cloves
Pinch ground nutmeg

Kofta kabobs are a traditional Middle Eastern dish. The spicing is rich
and fragrant but not hot. To start, use your fingers to thoroughly mix
together all of the ingredients in a large bowl. Next, on a flat surface,
such as a plastic cutting board, take a handful of the meat and either roll
it into a hot-dog shape about 6 inches long or roll it in the same shape

onto metal skewers. (Squared off or rectangular skewers work better than round.) Place the kabobs or skewers on a grill or the wire rack of a baking pan. (Precoat the wires with a little olive oil to prevent the meat from sticking.) Cooking times will vary, depending on your grill and oven, but the kabobs will most likely be cooked in 4 to 5 minutes.

THAI RED CURRY SEAFOOD STEW

(Serves 4)

1 tablespoon macadamia nut oil or coconut oil
2–3 cloves garlic, sliced thinly
½ cup cut-up baby asparagus stalks (trimmed and cut into 1-inch pieces)
½ cup sliced mushrooms
¼ cup thinly sliced red and green bell peppers
4 baby corn ears, cut in half
12-ounce can coconut milk (not lite)
1 tablespoon Thai Kitchen Green Curry Paste
½ teaspoon ground turmeric
¼ teaspoon red pepper flakes
½ pound shrimp, cleaned and deveined
½ pound firm white fish, such as tilapia, cut into 1-inch chunks
Optional: ½ teaspoon Thai Kitchen Fish Sauce (optional because it contains some sugar)
¼ cup fresh, tender basil leaves

Heat the oil in a deep skillet on high heat, and, when hot, sauté the garlic, asparagus, mushrooms, bell peppers, and corn. Slowly pour the coconut milk into the skillet, then add the curry paste, turmeric, and red pepper flakes. Using a spatula, thoroughly mix the paste into the coconut milk, while bringing it to a light boil. Add the shrimp and fish, stirring so that all of the seafood is covered by the coconut milk. Cover the skillet (use aluminum foil if you don't have a cover), turn the heat down to medium, and cook the stew for 15 minutes, stirring occasionally. Add the basil leaves and cook for about 1 minute more. Serve the stew with steamed cauliflower and brown or purple "Forbidden" rice.

Side Dishes

GREEN BEANS, MUSHROOMS, SHALLOTS, AND ALMONDS

(Serves 4)

½ pound fresh green beans, ends trimmed
2 teaspoons olive oil
2 shallots, chopped
¼ cup sliced chanterelle mushrooms*
¼ cup toasted almond slices or slivers
2 tablespoons fresh chopped cilantro
½ teaspoon dried Greek oregano (or 1 tablespoon chopped fresh)
Salt

Add some water to a large saucepan, and bring it to a boil. Add the green beans and cook them for 5 to 7 minutes. Drain the water and transfer the green beans to a large mixing bowl. Meanwhile, heat the oil on medium high in a small nonstick skillet. Add the shallots and mushrooms, and sauté for about 3 to 4 minutes (until the shallots soften). Add the shallots and mushrooms to the green beans. Add the almonds and cilantro, sprinkle everything with oregano and salt, and toss.

* *Note*: You can use fresh or dried and rehydrated chanterelle mushrooms.

BOK CHOY STIR-FRY

(Serves 2)

2 tablespoons olive oil
3 cloves garlic, minced
1 pound bok choy, rinsed, dried, and chopped
1 tablespoon tamari

Heat the oil in a large wok on medium-high heat. Sauté the garlic for about 1 minute, then add the bok choy and sauté until it's soft (about 5 to 10 minutes). Add the tamari, mix it thoroughly with the bok choy, and serve.

SNOW PEA STIR FRY
(Serves 2)

2 tablespoons olive oil
1 clove garlic, minced
1 pound snow peas, rinsed, dried
¼ cup pine nuts
1 tablespoon tamari

Heat the oil in a large wok on medium-high heat. Sauté the garlic for about 1 minute, then add the snow peas and sauté until some of the snow peas start to caramelize (about 5 minutes). Add the pine nuts and continue to sauté for another minute. Then add the tamari, mix it thoroughly with the snow peas, and serve.

STEAMED VEGETABLES
(Serves 2–4)

You don't need an expensive device to steam vegetables. Most supermarkets sell metal steamer baskets, which you can insert into a saucepan. Add enough water so that it just touches the bottom of the steamer. Add broccoli or cauliflower crowns to the steamer basket, and turn the heat on high to cook the vegetables for 8 to 10 minutes. If you want to steam carrots, use either baby carrots or cut larger carrots into small pieces, then place them in the steamer basket. Cook them on high heat for 10 to 15 minutes, until you can easily pierce the carrots with a fork.

MINT CHUTNEY
(Serves 4)

2 cups fresh mint leaves
½ cup cilantro leaves

1 tablespoon chopped Anaheim chili pepper (seeds removed);
   alternatively, for more hotness, 1 jalapeño pepper, seeds
   removed, chopped
½ cup chopped red onion
1 tablespoon garam masala spice blend
2 tablespoons fresh lemon juice
2 tablespoons or more water

Place all of the ingredients in a food processor or a blender and puree.
If the chutney is too thick, add a little more water (up to ½ cup total) to
thin it. Use this as a dipping sauce for tandoori chicken or for cooked
turkey or lamb chunks.

SAUTÉED FENNEL, OLIVES, AND RAISINS
(Serves 4)

2 fennel bulbs, cut into thin strips
1 tablespoon olive oil
2 tablespoons diced black olives
2 tablespoons organic Thompson raisins
Juice of 1 lemon

Remove and discard the green stems from the fennel bulbs before you
cut or shred them into thin strips. Heat the oil in a large wok. Sauté
the fennel strips until they are tender and start to caramelize, 15 to 30
minutes, depending on their thickness. Add the black olives and raisins,
reduce the heat to a simmer, and stir the ingredients together. Add the
lemon juice, stir, and serve.

BAKED ASPARAGUS WITH PANCETTA
(Serves 3)

12 ounces fresh asparagus spears
¼ red onion, thinly sliced
2 slices pancetta, diced
Extra-virgin olive oil

Cut off the woody 1-inch bottoms of the asparagus stems. Then use a vegetable peeler to remove the skin along the lower part of the stems. Lay the asparagus spears on a baking sheet. Arrange the onion slices and pancetta on top of the asparagus. Drizzle everything with extra-virgin olive oil. Bake the dish for 3 minutes at 400 degrees F. Use a spatula to flip the asparagus over, and bake it for another 3 minutes. Scoop up the onions and pancetta, and spread it on top of the asparagus when you serve the dish.

ROSEMARY CARROTS
(Serves 2)

8 ounces baby carrots or large carrots cut into ½-inch pieces
Extra-virgin olive oil
2 teaspoons fresh chopped or dried rosemary leaves

Clean and peel the carrots as necessary, and place them in a microwave-safe bowl. Drizzle extra-virgin olive oil over the carrots, and sprinkle the rosemary leaves over them. Microwave them at medium-high power for 4 minutes. The carrots will cook for 1 or 2 more minutes after being heated.

EXOTIC RICE
(Serves 4)

There are so many varieties of rice—brown, purple, red, and jasmine, to name just a few—that plain old white rice seems boring. One of the best sources of these and other rice varieties is your natural food store or www .lotusfoods.com. All of these types of rice take longer to cook than white rice does. For short- or long-grain brown rice, rinse 1 cup of rice under cold water and transfer it to a large saucepan. Add 1 cup of chicken or vegetable broth, plus 1 cup of water. Heat this on high until the water boils, then reduce the heat to a simmer for approximately 40 minutes. Remove the rice from the heat source and fluff it with a fork. Be careful not to overcook the rice. Follow the same steps with Lotus Foods' red, purple, or jasmine rice, but cook it for only 30 to 35 minutes.

ITALIAN-STYLE TOMATO SAUCE
(Serves 4)

This is an easy homemade sauce that you can use with pizza or chicken breasts, especially if you have used basil and oregano to season the chicken.

2 tablespoons extra-virgin olive oil
½ cup diced or chopped mild onions
2–3 garlic cloves, diced
1–3 cups tomato puree or sauce (from a can or a jar)
3–4 tablespoons tomato paste
1 teaspoon dried basil
1 teaspoon dried oregano
1 bay leaf
1 teaspoon honey
Sea salt
Pepper

Heat the oil in a 2-quart saucepan on medium heat. Next, add the onion and garlic, stir them occasionally, and cook until they are slightly soft. Add the tomato puree/sauce and tomato paste, along with the basil, oregano, bay leaf, and honey, and simmer everything, covered, for 40 minutes. Add the salt and pepper. You can freeze the sauce for later use with other recipes, such as Lamb Meatballs with Sauce (see the recipe on page 173).

Soup

HEARTY ASIAN-STYLE SOUP
(Serves 1–2)

1 handful uncooked kuzu pasta
1 tablespoon macadamia nut oil or other neutral cooking oil

2 garlic cloves, diced

1 tablespoon minced or grated ginger

1 to 2 ounces tofu, firm variety, cut into cubes

½ cup or so fresh sliced shiitake mushrooms, stems removed

16 ounces chicken, beef, or vegetable broth

1 cup chopped napa cabbage

3 tablespoons or so tamari

1–2 tablespoons sesame oil

1 scallion, thinly sliced

In a saucepan, heat enough water to boil a handful of kuzu pasta. (Alternatively, use 100 percent buckwheat soba noodles, both available from www.edenfoods.com.) Cook the kuzu pasta per the package instructions, reducing the boiling water to a simmer for 8 minutes. Meanwhile, put the macadamia nut oil in a separate saucepan on medium-high heat. Add the garlic, ginger, and tofu, and sauté for 1 minute. Toss in the shiitake mushrooms, and sauté for another minute. Pour in the broth, bring it to a boil, and then reduce it to a simmer. Stir in the chopped napa cabbage and tamari. When the kuzu pasta is cooked, drain off the water and add the pasta to the broth with vegetables. Add the sesame oil. Allow everything to simmer for 1 or 2 more minutes , transfer the soup to a bowl, sprinkle on the scallion, and serve.

---

quick tip
Choosing a High-Quality Chicken Broth

Read the fine print on the list of ingredients, and you might be shocked by what some companies add to their chicken broth. Certain brands have monosodium glutamate, sugar, or huge amounts of salt. My top recommendations are for Pacific (also sold under the Trader Joe's label), Health Valley, and Imagine. Most of these companies also sell beef and vegetable broths.

CHICKEN RICE SOUP

Leftover bones and some chicken meat
1 medium-size red or sweet onion, diced
3 stalks celery hearts, diced
2–3 large carrots, cleaned and sliced
1 teaspoon dried thyme*
2 bay leaves
1 teaspoon fresh ground black pepper
Filtered water
1 cup cooked brown rice
Sea salt

You'll need a stockpot (at least 6 inches deep) for this recipe. You will also want four to six plastic containers to freeze the soup for later use.

Use a leftover chicken carcass. Remove and discard as much of the chicken skin as possible. Place the bones in the stock pot. Add the onion, celery, carrot, thyme, bay leaves, and ground pepper. Add enough cold water to cover the chicken. Bring the water to a boil, place the cover a little ajar so that some of the water can evaporate and reduce the soup, and then simmer the soup for 3 hours. Turn off the heat, cover the pot tightly, and allow it to cool (such as for several hours or overnight). When it cools, put the pot in the refrigerator.

After it's cool, use a large spoon to skim the hardened fat off the top of the broth. Pull off any meat from the carcass and return the meat to the soup. Discard the bones. Use a slotted spoon to sift through the soup for small bones, joints, or gristle, and throw them out.

Now put some of the cooked brown rice in the plastic containers. Use a ladle to transfer the soup from the pot to the containers, but leave a little room for the soup to expand when it freezes. Place the containers in your freezer and date them. When you're ready to have the soup, allow it to at least partially defrost before you transfer it to a small saucepan and heat it. Add sea salt.

*Note: Do not add thyme if the chicken was originally seasoned with tandoori spice mix.

SIMPLE SQUASH SOUP
(Serves 2)

1 butternut squash
Olive oil
2 cups chicken or vegetable broth
Sour cream
Dried sage

Cut the butternut squash in half, scoop it out, and discard the seeds. Lightly coat the exposed flesh with a small amount of olive oil, place the two halves flesh-side down on a baking dish, and bake them at 350 degrees F for 1 hour. Alternatively, buy cubed, ready-to-cook butternut squash, and follow the microwave directions to cook it until it's soft (typically, 10 to 15 minutes on high). Scoop out the cooked squash and place it in a blender with the chicken or vegetable broth (a good organic variety, such as Pacific brand). Blend until everything is a liquid. Transfer this to a saucepan, heat the soup on medium heat, and serve. Consider adding a dollop of sour cream, and sprinkle on a little dried sage.

Sample Two-Week Meal Plan

I encourage you to look at menu plans as idea generators, not as a rigid schedule that requires you to eat certain foods on certain days. As I mentioned earlier, eating a little protein for breakfast is fundamental if you want to maintain steady energy levels later in the day. You can certainly switch around lunches and dinners and reheat leftovers to save time. For example, many dinner leftovers work well when they're chopped and mixed with scrambled eggs. It's also easy to take leftovers to work and reheat them in a toaster oven or a microwave oven. An asterisk (*) indicates that the recipe is in this book. Many of the other recipes can be found in my previous books and cookbooks and on the Internet.

Part of my approach to cooking is to make an initial investment in time that provides a "return on my investment," in that leftovers save time for several subsequent meals. With that in mind, make part of your

Sunday (or another day of your choosing) a cooking and food-prep day. Start by preparing enough scrambled eggs and sautéed vegetables so that you can store leftovers in ramekins for quick reheating on Monday and Tuesday morning. Likewise, roast a chicken or a turkey breast on Sunday evening, which can provide leftovers for several days.

Day 1: Sunday
Breakfast Scrambled Eggs and Sautéed Vegetables*
Lunch Ceviche*
Dinner Roast Turkey Breast with Rubbed Sage*

Day 2: Monday
Breakfast Reheat Scrambled Eggs and Sautéed Vegetables*
Lunch Curried Turkey Salad* with Simple Green Side Salad*
Dinner Turkey Tacos*

Day 3: Tuesday
Breakfast Reheat Scrambled Eggs and Sautéed Vegetables *
Lunch Curried Turkey Salad* with apple slices
Dinner Mediterranean-Style Pan-Fried Chicken Breasts, with vegetables

Day 4: Wednesday
Breakfast Steel-Cut Oatmeal* with blueberries
Lunch Lamb Burgers*
Dinner Rotisserie Chicken on the Run*

Day 5: Thursday
Breakfast Steel-Cut Oatmeal* with diced apple and cinnamon
Lunch Greek Salad and Dressing*
Dinner Tandoori Shrimp*

Day 6: Friday
Breakfast Easy Poached Eggs* with fruit on the side
Lunch Roast beef and cheese slices, with apple
Dinner Buckwheat Noodle Pasta with Rich Red Sauce*

Day 7: Saturday
Breakfast   Easy Poached Eggs Danish-Style Smørrebrød*
Lunch   Simple Tomato and Mozzarella Cheese Salad*
Dinner   Marinated Chicken Breasts*

Day 8: Sunday
Breakfast   Chicken and Avocado Omelet
Lunch   Green Salad with Grilled Chicken*
Dinner   Roasted Whole Chicken,* with vegetables

Day 9: Monday
Breakfast   Scrambled Eggs with Ground Turkey*
Lunch   Defrosted Chicken Rice Soup*
Dinner   Sautéed scallops and shrimp in olive oil, basil, and
              oregano

Day 10: Tuesday
Breakfast   Steel-Cut Oatmeal* with Fruit Salad* on the side
Lunch   Vietnamese chicken spring rolls
Dinner   Thai Red Curry Seafood Stew*

Day 11: Wednesday
Breakfast   Simple Scrambled Egg*
Lunch   Greek-style gyro meat on salad
Dinner   Poached salmon with crème sauce, with vegetables

Day 12: Thursday
Breakfast   German-Style Antipasto (Meat and Cheese) Plate*
Lunch   Super-Savvy Light Deli Lunch*
Dinner   Salad with flaked poached salmon (leftover from previ-
              ous night), oil and vinegar dressing

Day 13: Friday
Breakfast   Simple Scrambled Egg* with a side of fresh fruit
Lunch   Chicken Caesar salad (sans croutons)
Dinner   Chicken Piccata with Vegetables

Day 14: Saturday

Breakfast   Cheese Omelet with a Hint of Rosemary*
Lunch   Simple Squash Soup* and Simple Green Side Salad*
Dinner   Sea Scallops in Butter and Wine Sauce*

chapter 9

Reducing Stress to Ease Your Fatigue

In chapter 1, I explained how chronic stress formed the first circle of fatigue and had a powerful bearing on the other circles, as well as on the Fatigue Syndrome. Chronic stress leads to negative changes in your eating habits, hormone levels, risk of disease, and the rate at which your body and mind age. To reduce your fatigue and improve your energy levels, it is essential that you recognize the major stresses in your life and find ways to pare down or manage them.

Unfortunately, it's often difficult to think clearly about managing stress when you feel stressed. Part of the reason is that adrenaline, your fight-or-flight hormone, prompts the brain to make rapid decisions, rather than contemplative and thoughtful ones. After all, in your ancient biology, running for your life and dodging a predator demanded split-second decisions, and any hesitation would have meant being eaten.

In today's world, stress makes you more reactive than proactive in your thinking and actions. In addition, your breathing becomes shallow, so the brain does not receive optimal amounts of oxygen, which can also affect your thinking processes. You end up getting carried along by stress, as if it were an undertow, and any semblance of balance in your life drowns. This lack of balance impedes your ability to rest, fight fatigue, and recoup your energy. Cortisol, the other primary stress hormone, actually destroys brain cells, impairing memory and cognitive function, increasing the risk of adrenal exhaustion, and multiplying your long-term odds of developing Alzheimer's disease.

Teach Yourself to Disconnect from Stress

How can you protect yourself from, or at least blunt the effect of, the stresses that surround you? There is a lesson to be learned from the way parents sometimes impose a "time-out" on unruly children. The time-out serves as a reset button, isolating a child from part of his or her environment and creating a several-minute break to help the child calm down. You might think you're more self-aware than a child is, but you actually aren't, whenever you feel stressed. You're simply wrapped up in responding to the stress.

You can, however, cultivate a psychological "reset button" to remind yourself to take a break when you feel too stressed—in effect, to give yourself a brief time-out. The important point here is really twofold: first, learning to recognize when you're overly stressed and, second, interrupting your stress response for at least a few minutes. You'll feel better, and you'll function more effectively as well.

I recommend that you use one of several techniques, choosing those that you are most comfortable with.

Breathing   Remembering to breathe deeply becomes especially important during the shallow breathing that typically occurs when you feel stressed. The nice thing about breathing exercises is that you can do them anywhere, such as at your desk or in a car. Take three or four slow and very deep breaths. Doing so can ease feelings of anxiety that are commonly associated with being stressed.

Meditation   A brief period of meditation can help restore a sense of calmness and improve your mental clarity when you return to the task at hand. Meditation does not need to have any religious overtones, although prayer is often a form of meditation. Sit in a chair, with the backs of your hands resting either on your knees or on the chair's arms. Close your eyes, try to relax your back and arm muscles, breathe deeply, and focus your thoughts on a peaceful experience, such as lying on a beach or listening to a classical music concert.

Yoga   As with meditation, you can adopt some simple yoga practices to help you disengage from stress, and you don't have to twist your body into difficult positions. Sit cross-legged on the floor, or simply sit on the floor if you cannot cross your legs. Close your eyes, breathe deeply, and focus your thoughts on a single tranquil experience from your past. Do this for a minute or two. If you would like a more structured but relatively uncomplicated approach to yoga, consider visiting yogafordepression.com and buying a copy of this CD: *LifeForce Yoga Bhavana: Say Yes to Yourself—A Guided Relaxation Experience with Amy Weintraub*. Simply listening to Amy's soothing voice can help erase your stress.

Stretching   Muscles of the back tend to tighten up when you're stressed, and a simple stretch or two can loosen them up. Sit on the floor, bend one leg to raise the knee, lean forward to the knee, and wrap your arms around it. Hold this position for about 30 seconds. Stretch out that leg, and follow the same steps using your other leg. Alternatively, lie on your back with your legs outstretched. Raise one knee as close to your chest as possible, wrap your arms around it, and hold this position for about 30 seconds. Relax the leg and repeat, using your other leg.

Walking   The key here is not to go for a long walk but only for a short one to distract you from your stress. If you're at work, take five minutes to walk down the hallways. If you're at home, walk around the house or up and down the stairs. You can also walk to the bathroom — we often forget to do this when we're stressed. While walking, be sure to let your eyes fall on objects that are a different focal length from those you normally look at. For example, if you do most of your work at a desk or a computer, look into the distance while you walk. While refocusing your eyes, you'll also refocus your brain.

Think inwardly   Allow yourself to be alone with your own thoughts. Some people seem to do almost anything to avoid being alone with their thoughts. They've got to be on the phone, listening to the radio, watching television, or listening to their MP3 player. The problem? The radio, the television, and the phone can add to your stress, and turning them off can actually reduce your stress. Often, television and radio shows are little more than distracting background noise, when a quiet period would be much more relaxing. Television stations boost the volume during commercials, and louder sounds are more stressful than soft sounds or the absence of sounds. Consider some possible alternatives, such as reading a book or a magazine or simply letting your thoughts wander for a while.

How to Reduce Time Stress

So many of our day-to-day stresses boil down to a single issue: not having enough time to do everything the world asks of us. Between work and home, most of us have plenty to do, and there are only so many hours in a day, even when we try to stretch out our waking hours to the point of fatigue. I have some suggestions for reducing time stress and helping you overcome the Fatigue Syndrome.

Maintain or reestablish your personal boundaries. Stressful situations tend to overwhelm your personal boundaries, and often you're not as vigilant as you could be in maintaining these boundaries. When your boundaries dissolve, stressful situations start to chip away at your time and energy.

The concept of personal boundaries is a frequent topic in many relationship books. In so many ways, boundaries are about protecting your personal space, your integrity, and sometimes your body. When a woman says no to a man, she is establishing a personal boundary. In terms of day-to-day stresses, boundaries are something like the territorial waters that surround nations with coastlines. You own them, but you have to guard them to discourage others from violating what are essentially your buffer zones. When you don't maintain these boundaries, you essentially allow others to invade your space.

As much of the working world moved from a forty-hour week to a global 24/7 economy, various communications technologies (such as e-mail and cell phones) encouraged work to cross our personal boundaries and make incursions into our evenings, weekends, and vacations. Granted, many of us have to occasionally work on an evening or a weekend. But when we regularly permit coworkers or clients to contact us about work in the evenings and on weekends—or if we take the time to respond to their requests—we end up sacrificing some of the personal time that is essential for recharging our energy.

How can we limit these incursions? It helps to remember that there is a time and a place for everything, and checking e-mails or posting comments on Facebook until midnight will rob you of sleep. Similarly, a ringing phone or a text mail chime rarely requires an immediate response—it's often better to simply stay focused on what you are currently doing. After all, how much fun is it to have a ringing phone (think telemarketers) interrupt a relaxing meal or sex?

Relationship Stresses at Work and at Home

Nearly all conflicts or perceived conflicts (such as those we fabricate where none really exist) revolve around our dealings with other people, and these conflicts wear us down. The most common stress-generating aspects of work are bosses, coworkers, deadlines, workload, office politics, and commuting. Many people use the workplace to act out their inner turmoil and in the process make life difficult for other people. Relationships at home can also be riddled with stress. Some conflicts are inevitable between spouses, parents and children, and in-laws, but half of all marriages in the United States end in divorce, which is a sign of the seriousness of certain conflicts.

One fundamental cause of relationship conflicts is the desire to control another person, such as a family member or a coworker. It's nearly impossible to control the acts of another person, and attempting to do so almost always breeds resentment and resistance. Many of these control issues are related to another person not doing what you want him or her to do, although expectations of behavior are not always clearly stated. Both trying to control another person and being controlled by another person are stress generators.

Sometimes people are simply too tired to discuss and sincerely negotiate important issues and differences. Other times, they have difficulty coming up with the right words, or they overreact to what the other person says. Unless these conflicts are resolved, either by discussion or by simply giving the other person some "space," small resentments will grow until they become irreconcilable differences. Along the way, many people simply decide that they've become worn out by the relationship.

Tips to Reduce Work and Home Stress

It takes an effort to decrease the interpersonal conflicts and resentments that lie at the root of almost all types of stress. If relationship stress at work or at home is part of your life, ratcheting down the tension is essential if you want to boost your energy and change the aspects of your life that contribute to the Fatigue Syndrome.

Give up control. It's an adage among psychological counselors that the only person you can control is yourself. Yet so many people continue to try, usually unsuccessfully, to control situations or other people. They may exert some measure of control through intimidation. Yet if they could only discuss the problem without name calling or arm twisting, this would often lead to a constructive resolution or compromise. Speaking directly and calmly also saves a lot of energy that might otherwise be spent in frustration or argument. Granted, this type of discussion requires skill, calmness, and carefully modulated words to avoid blaming the other person. For example, you might say something like, "I really get annoyed when you don't replace an empty roll of toilet paper. I would appreciate it if you would replace it next time."

Get unstuck. Many people are "stuck" in life—essentially motionless, unable to change or move forward. They may suffer in a draining job or a bad marriage but remain unsure of what to do to improve their situation. I have had my share of difficult times, but in each case, I eventually resolved to find a way to deal with them. Once I accepted a job with a small magazine, only to find on the first day that it was not for me. On the second day I resigned, and two administrative assistants confessed that they had wondered how long I would stay. Apparently, I was not the first editor to quickly leave. We had a good laugh together before I left. It's all too easy to become habituated to a bad situation because it might seem better than an unknown alternative. It is far better to deal with the unknown and build our self-esteem and personal strength.

Don't take it personally. Some people say nasty things or honk their horns at you, but their frustration and rage may not be your fault. They may simply be frustrated or angry. You can ease some of the stress in your life by not taking everything that other people say or do personally. Criticisms and honking car horns are often motivated by issues that have nothing to do with you. If you let yourself get riled up, you'll get stressed and eventually feel worn down.

Don't overreact. Try listening to a coworker or a family member without being reactive and getting into an argument. That's the sage advice of psychologist Michael P. Nichols, Ph.D., in *The Lost Art of Listening*. You always have a choice between reacting, responding calmly, or walking away, although these choices often escape people. Sometimes, deciding not to be reactive requires a tremendous amount of patience. The other person may try to bait you to engage in an adrenaline-stimulating argument that no one will win. If you do react, the disagreement will likely escalate into a destructive, take-no-prisoners battle. (Think of the knock-down, drag-out family feuds in the film *The Godfather*.) None of what I suggest means that you have to agree with the criticisms. Engaging in a nonreactive dialogue means keeping the conversation civil, discussing differences of opinion calmly instead of yelling, forgiving a poor choice of words, and trying to understand what's annoying the other person.

Susan Finds That Optimism Prevails over Stress

Susan, a friend of mine, is one of the most upbeat, optimistic, and energetic people I've ever known. A few years ago, she left a satisfying, high-profile job for one in which she could help other people and demonstrate her true creativity as a publicist.

She ended up getting the job from hell. Her new boss was controlling and abusive, and Susan's enthusiasm gave way to feelings of hurt and despair. One day, when I happened to visit her at work, she broke down and cried. I knew that something had to change.

In these circumstances, many people would look for another job, and so did Susan. Yet she ended up doing something that most others would consider risky. She simply quit her job to give herself some time to heal from an abusive situation and to explore different options. Within a year, she had devoted herself to photography, beginning with occasional assignments and building up contacts and an impressive portfolio. Ever the optimist, Susan's passion for photography became her next job, one that she relished and that easily earned her the respect of clients. In the process, she turned what could have been numbing fatigue into inexhaustible energy in her work.

Downtime and Vacations

A study by Oxford Health Plans found that one in every five American workers does not use all of his or her earned vacation time, usually because the person has too much work to do. In other words, people who need vacations the most don't take them. Other people avoid going on vacations because they fear that they'll return to even more work.

Whether people are voluntary or involuntary workaholics, they suffer serious consequences from not taking time off. An article in the *American Journal of Epidemiology* found that women who did not take vacations during a twenty-five-year period were more likely to suffer a heart attack or die from any cause, compared with women who did take vacations. It's simply another path to feeling run down.

Having downtime in the evenings and on weekends provides a period to recover from the stress of work and maintain balance in one's life as a whole. With that extra time, you can read a book, go to a movie, pursue hobbies, attend a sports event or a concert, or just have a good time with family and friends. Those social ties are especially important, because they are associated with people having a lower risk of disease and death. Social activities can also help reenergize you.

Make the Time

You can makes excuses for not taking a day off or a vacation, or you can make the time. It's a choice. If you live in a city, odds are that there are plenty of social events in the evenings and on weekends that you could attend. You don't have to go out more than once a week, but the intellectual and emotional stimulation of getting away from both work and home can have a profound effect on your biochemistry, breaking your normal routines and energizing you.

Take a vacation—after all, you've earned it! Here's how I do it: If I'm arranging a business trip and going someplace interesting, I'll usually add a day or two for personal activities, such as visiting art museums, looking for interesting things to photograph, or simply taking long walks. If I'm planning a vacation, I try to keep my itinerary fairly loose, typically reserving flights, a hotel room, and a car but keeping my day-to-day activities flexible and spontaneous. I might have a list of things to do, but my schedule could shift from day to day, for no reason other than the weather.

I understand that for some people, planning an actual vacation can be a daunting task. Although I'm comfortable with the unfamiliar, an unstructured travel style may be stressful for some people. The key, then, is to plan a vacation that relieves, rather than causes, stress. If planning the logistics seems overwhelming, work through a travel agent. (In fact, most major airlines will help you plan an entire trip for a very modest fee.) Decide what kind of vacation you want: exploring a new city, embarking on an outdoor adventure, or hanging around the pool at a resort. Take the time—after all, someone is paying you to go on vacation.

Time Shifting

Even the best job and work environment can rob you of energy if you happen to work the night shift. Night workers cross a wide range of professions and include factory workers, overseas airline crews, police officers, firemen, doctors, and nurses. People who work at night have a greater risk of developing cancer, heart disease, and infections. No wonder their hours are sometimes called the graveyard shift.

Although some of us might seem nocturnal in our habits, being more alert or creative at night, we're basically diurnal creatures. Night workers fight their biology, and they suffer the consequences, such as fatigue that is comparable to jet lag. Their body clocks typically remain mixed up for at least another day as they segue from working at night to being more active during the day. Then, just as they have started to readjust to a diurnal schedule, they go back to work at night again.

Take the case of Mary, who worked nights as a nurse for many years but no longer does. She was tired all of the time and felt as if she had no good-quality downtime before she had to go back to work. Her reflexes and thinking processes were essentially those of someone who was drunk, an effect that has been borne out by scientific studies. "It certainly affected my marriage," she recalled. "My husband and I couldn't do things together because he had a lot of energy and I didn't."

What happens to the bodies of night workers? Normally, the pineal gland starts to secrete the sleep-inducing hormone melatonin in the evening. To stay awake and to suppress melatonin levels, many night workers drink coffee or other caffeinated beverages (or eat chocolate, which contains caffeine and other brain-stimulating chemicals). Caffeine prompts the release of adrenaline, which helps promote alertness, and the liver releases sugar for additional energy. Yet the suppression of a normal melatonin cycle has long-term consequences. Melatonin helps prevent cancer and heart disease, it has antioxidant benefits, and it can also serve as a brain chemical that helps create a mellow mood. If you suppress melatonin, you're asking for sleep disorders, fatigue, and any number of health problems.

Night workers may also have a higher-than-normal risk of developing adrenal exhaustion. As they gear up to work nights, their daily cortisol pattern reverses itself. Normally, cortisol levels are highest in the morning and then decline in the afternoon and the evening. In night workers, cortisol levels tend to be highest in the evening. When adrenal exhaustion develops, cortisol levels drop during the entire day, and people feel completely wiped out—a sign that they may be suffering from the Fatigue Syndrome.

A related and uncomfortable shift in our circadian, or daily biological, rhythms occurs in the spring when most people move their clocks one hour ahead. The "spring ahead" leads to the loss of an hour of sleep, and people feel this loss of sleep for at least a few days after the time change. The "fall behind" is no fun, either; we may gain an hour of sleep, but then we end up commuting home in the dark and feeling disoriented and tired. Jet lag also affects our circadian rhythms, especially when we fly across more than one time zone, such as from coast to coast or overseas. If you fly from Chicago to London, you'll arrive around 8 a.m., but your body clock is probably somewhere around midnight.

Easing the Stress of Night Work

Paying close attention to your eating habits and taking two types of nutritional supplements may lessen, though not completely eliminate, some of the negative consequences of jet lag and working nights.

> *Eating habits*   Flying through multiple time zones stresses your circadian rhythm, but eating high-carbohydrate (including high-sugar) foods worsens the inevitable fatigue. That's because blood sugar fluctuations alone can make you feel tired. The same is true of night-shift workers, who try to stay alert when their bodies would prefer to be asleep. Eating higher protein meals (such as fish and chicken) and high-fiber vegetables, while avoiding sugary and starchy foods, can stabilize your blood sugar and energy levels. If you're planning to fly, adopt this eating pattern at least several days before flying.

Melatonin Supplements of this hormone are available without a prescription at most health food stores and pharmacies. Melatonin can promote a very restful sleep when taken one to two hours before bedtime. The effective dose can range considerably among individuals. I recommend starting at a very low dose, such as 250 to 500 mcg (0.25 to 0.5 mg) for a couple of days. If this amount does not cause drowsiness, increase it to 1 mg, then to 2 mg, and then to 3 mg. Most people don't need more than 3 mg before going to sleep, but you can safely go up to 5 mg. Don't drive in the evening after taking melatonin. If you're planning to fly, start to take melatonin a couple of days before you travel—but take 250 to 500 mcg at what would be an early evening hour at your destination.

Probiotics People who work nights are more susceptible to getting infections and other illnesses. Probiotic supplements contain "good bacteria" that support those that normally inhabit your digestive tract, and these bacteria release compounds that enhance the immune system's ability to fight infection. In a Swedish study of night-shift workers, none of the people consuming probiotic supplements called in sick, whereas one-fourth of those taking placebos did call in. Various types of probiotic supplements are sold in health food stores.

Depression, Post-Traumatic Stress Disorder, and Fatigue

Persistent feelings of depression, anxiety, or post-traumatic stress disorder can be major contributors to fatigue and the Fatigue Syndrome. I've written about these conditions in my book *The Food-Mood Solution*.

Depression

Depression comes in many forms and has many different causes, some psychological and others nutritional and biochemical in origin. Yet depressed energy levels are often associated with a depressed mood.

Feelings of depression are a normal emotion during periods of grief. In many ways, depression is part of a rite of passage, such as after the death of a spouse. Feelings of depression may last several months, after which time the survivor starts to shed feelings of sadness and redefine his or her life.

Other psychosocial issues can also precipitate depression. These issues may relate to feeling "stuck" in an unsatisfying job or marriage. Although this type of depression is now often treated with medications, it makes far more sense to resolve the life issues that underlie the depression, perhaps by making changes in one's life. By resolution, I don't mean that a person always has to change jobs or get divorced. Rather, it may entail some degree of acceptance or emotional detachment regarding the job or renewing a commitment to the marriage.

When psychosocial issues result in depression, the emotions prompt changes in one's brain chemistry. These changes involve alterations in neurotransmitters, the chemicals that regulate mood. Dietary lapses can reinforce the changes because neurotransmitter activity depends on nutrients. In some people, inherited genetic "weaknesses" can interfere with the activity of nutrients and neurotransmitters and increase the risk of depression. Sometimes nutritional deficiencies lead to depression, particularly when there is no obvious cause of the psychological entropy. For example, protein and B vitamins are necessary ingredients in the formation of neurotransmitters, and contemporary diets are often low in these nutrients.

Physicians work from a checklist of clinical symptoms that can point to depression. The simplest and clearest definition of depression is this: sadness plus hopelessness (the feeling that life will not get better). Sometimes anger is a sign of depression. Other common signs include a lack of motivation, reduced interest in activities that were previously enjoyable, feelings of worthlessness and guilt, weight gain, fantasies about death or suicide, and, of course, fatigue.

Post-Traumatic Stress Disorder

The emotional trauma of war has been understood for thousands of years, but it wasn't until 1980 that the third edition of the *Diagnostic and Statistical Manual of Mental Disorders* (DSM-III) used the term *post-traumatic stress disorder* (PTSD). Until then, this type of psychological trauma was sometimes called a stress-response syndrome or a nervous breakdown.

The symptoms of PTSD often include depression and anxiety, reexperiencing the original trauma through flashbacks and nightmares, noise sensitivity, hypervigilance, irritability and anger, feeling emotionally numbed, or having panic attacks. PTSD occurs in approximately one-third of the soldiers who have been in combat, but psychological trauma can affect many other people. People who have been abused as children, have been raped, and have witnessed acts of terrorism often suffer from PTSD. A study in the *Journal of the American Medical Association* reported that sixty-one thousand people who saw the collapse of the World Trade Center towers in 2001 were experiencing PTSD at least six years later.

Intense stress prompts the secretion of large amounts of cortisol, and this hormone seems to imprint stressful events on the brain. Conventional treatments for PTSD include talk therapy, medications, and sometimes "exposure therapy" to replay the experience and dull the person's responses to memories of it. Inexplicably, most doctors seem to ignore the role of adrenal exhaustion in PTSD. (Please refer back to chapter 3.) In addition, nutritional therapies are commonly overlooked, but several nutritional supplements can help reduce the depression and anxiety associated with PTSD. I discuss these supplements in the next section.

Some Solutions for Depression and PTSD

There are so many causes of depression and PTSD that it is difficult to suggest any single solution. Yet certain specific lifestyle changes and nutritional supplements can frequently lead to improvement, and an increase in energy often follows.

Lifestyle changes   I sometimes use the French word *ennui* (pronounced ahn-wee) to describe depression. Ennui refers to an apathy, a weariness, or a dissatisfaction with life, combined with a loss of interest in activities. Part of the psychosocial response, then, should be to find new meaning in life or new activities to pursue. After you identify the vacuum in your life or the source of your depression or anxiety, the next step is to consider the options for improving your life.

Some people successfully resolve their depression through stronger religious faith or a nonreligious spiritual practice. Spiritual practices can take many different forms, such as traditional religion and prayer, spending time in nature, meditating, or practicing yoga. My friend and professional colleague Amy Weintraub cured her own deep depression through the mental and physical discipline of yoga. She developed LifeForce Yoga, became one of the leading yoga teachers in the United States, and wrote *Yoga for Depression* to describe her experiences and provide a path for other people to follow. As Amy is quick to point out, considerable scientific research supports the role of yoga, meditation, and breathing practices on mood and cognition.

Many depressed people lack a physical or emotional connection with other people. Physically touching or being touched by another person has a profound effect on biochemistry and mood. If you are in a relationship with another person, cuddling, touch, and pillow talk can strengthen the interpersonal bond and lessen feelings of depression. Essentially, touch provides a tangible connection with another human being, easing the feelings of isolation that are often associated with depression. Another option is a therapeutic non-sexual massage, which can also have a very positive effect on your mood. Similarly, the Bio-Touch technique (www.justtouch.com/default.shtml) uses a series of light, butterfly-like touches to enhance mood and reduce pain.

Laughing can be profoundly beneficial for your mood and overall health. Researchers at the Positive Psychology Center at the University of Pennsylvania, Philadelphia, have been researching the qualities that make people happy. Their efforts reflect a major shift in the fields of psychology and psychiatry, which have long focused on behavioral and mood problems. People who laugh (but not at the expense of other people) are less likely to die of heart disease and other health problems. They have stronger immune systems and are better able to cope with stress.

You might wonder what humor and laughter have to do with energy levels. It's simple: being in a good mood is the antithesis of depression and, because of that, is more likely to be associated with higher energy levels. Even tired people can usually find the energy to laugh. In one study, researchers showed that laughter improved blood vessel tone in a way similar to that of a healthy diet or exercise. Laughter also serves as a release for anxiety.

Dietary supplements Nearly all mood issues are influenced at least in part by dietary habits. Low intake of the B vitamins and omega-3 fish oils can increase your susceptibility to depression, anxiety, and PTSD. Many scientific studies have shown that nutritional supplements, sold at health food stores and pharmacies, can have significant benefits in enhancing mood. These supplements work by supporting the normal biochemistry of the brain.

- A high-potency B-complex or high-potency multivitamin (containing the B vitamins) supplement provides broad nutritional support for healthy brain chemistry. By enhancing normal brain chemistry and nerve function, the B vitamins have an antidepressant and antianxiety effect. Look for approximately 50 mg of vitamins B_1, B_2, and B_3—amounts of the other B vitamins should fall into place.
- Omega-3 fish oils contain healthy fats that every cell in your body requires. In the brain, omega-3s enhance the ability of neurons to communicate with one another. Many studies have shown that fish oil supplements can relieve depression, anxiety, and irritability. Take two to three capsules daily.

- 5-HTP (5-hydroxytryptophan) is the immediate precursor to serotonin, a neurotransmitter that has antidepressant and antianxiety benefits. Try taking 50 to 200 mg of 5-HTP daily, in divided doses and at least one hour away from meals.
- The herb Saint-John's-wort has an exceptional track record for the treatment of depression. Take 300 mg three times daily (for a total of 900 mg). You can double the amount for severe depression.
- Chromium picolinate supplements are particularly beneficial for people who are depressed and overweight. Chromium picolinate may work by stabilizing blood sugar, which reduces appetite and also improves mood.

If you are currently taking antidepressant or antianxiety medications, do not stop taking them. Instead, ask your physician to monitor and help guide you as you transition to one of the previously mentioned natural therapies. These supplements have fewer side effects than prescription drugs do, and studies show that they are at least as effective.

chapter 10

Learning to Sleep Well

Millions of people share a similar experience: they go through the day feeling tired, yet they can't get a restful night's sleep. When the alarm goes off in the morning, they remain in denial for a few minutes, then drag themselves out of bed, stoke themselves with caffeine and a brisk shower, and trudge off to work. Welcome once again to the Fatigue Syndrome.

All five circles of fatigue can interfere with your sleep. Stress-related anxiety and worries can stimulate the brain and leave you tossing and turning throughout the night. Consuming caffeine in the afternoon and the evening is a common cause of insomnia. Hormone imbalances, including hot flashes, can wake women in the middle of the night. Some health problems, such as an enlarged prostate and associated urinary problems, can awaken men to go to the bathroom, making it difficult for them to return to sleep. And a lot of older folks complain of not getting enough hours of sleep.

As obvious as it might seem, many people forget that enjoying sufficient restful sleep is de rigueur for maintaining optimal energy levels and mental focus. Your body requires sleep to recover and rejuvenate. If you don't sleep well, you will age faster than normal, and your risk of becoming overweight and developing diabetes, heart disease, and cancer will skyrocket. Ominously, a lack of sleep may lead to long-term or permanent changes in biochemistry and brain architecture. And, frequent sleep loss makes it more difficult for you to recover by getting extra sleep.

Even though most people spend about one-third of their lives sleeping, scientists aren't completely sure why humans (and other animals) sleep. Sleep is essential for learning and memory. According to a recent article in *Science News*, people who have a nap with an REM (rapid eye movement) cycle, in which most dreams occur, do about 40 percent better on creative tests, compared with people who don't nap or don't have an REM cycle while napping. Studies have shown that people who sleep six hours or fewer each night are less likely to be efficient workers, eat healthy foods, exercise, or have sex, compared with people who sleep eight or more hours nightly. Yet such findings beg the question: is poor sleep the consequence or the cause of an unhealthy lifestyle? The question may never really be answered, but we do know that sleep problems are definitely intertwined with other bad habits. Fix one of the issues, and the others may start to improve.

Sleep isn't only for resting, though. During sleep, the immune system renews itself—hence the common recommendation for rest during illnesses. In addition, genes involved in the manufacture of large molecules, such as proteins and hormones, are more active during sleep. And, of course, psychoanalysts and others place great importance on the symbolism of dreams. Sometimes dream content is significant, but often dreams are little more than the brain shuffling through experiences the way a poker player shuffles a deck of cards.

What Interferes with Your Sleep

The most common causes of sleep problems are usually related to the five circles of fatigue. I'll briefly review these sleep disrupters, then suggest both lifestyle changes and supplements that can safely enhance the quality of your sleep and help you overcome the Fatigue Syndrome.

Lifestyle stress   People in the United States and other Western nations sleep about one hour less per night compared with people a hundred years ago. Of course, a lot has changed in the lives of people during the last century. One is that electric lighting has become far more common, which enables us to get more accomplished instead of sleeping. We also have businesses that run 24/7 and compete internationally, so, in many respects, much of the planet is lit up and working all of the time.

Then, at home, there's dinner to cook, laundry to be done, and bills to be paid. Between work and home life, there's almost always something that must be done, and this virtually nonstop activity wears us down, leaving us tired. And when we can relax at home, we are practically addicted to the television, e-mail, and texting—so that we end up feeling overstimulated and stressed and often stay up too late (somewhat like a child who doesn't know when to lie down and go to sleep). All of these activities contribute to stress, and our response to stress almost always includes greater anxiety. When we are anxious, it's difficult for us to calm down enough to sleep restfully.

Eating habits   Consuming caffeine in the afternoon and the evening can rev up the central nervous system, making it difficult to sleep. Many people add alcohol to the mix, which has a depressant effect, but when combined with caffeine, it gives the body mixed up-and-down signals. In addition, heartburn, often caused by consuming soft drinks or processed foods in the evening, can disrupt sleep.

Hormones   Low or fluctuating hormone levels can directly or indirectly rob us of energy. Many middle-aged women and their physicians attribute low energy levels to the decreased estrogen levels of perimenopause and menopause, but often the cause is low levels of adrenal and thyroid hormones, elevated insulin levels (a sign of prediabetes), or a combination of abnormal hormone levels. Hot flashes are one chief symptom of perimenopause, and hot flashes often disrupt women's sleep and increase their feelings of tiredness the next day.

Illnesses   Many illnesses also disrupt sleep. In men, benign prostate enlargement leads to urinary symptoms, including a powerful desire to urinate. When this happens in the middle of the night, it interrupts sleep and inevitably results in feelings of tiredness. Benign prostate enlargement can usually be helped with lycopene supplements, which are made from a tomato extract. Being overweight or having type 2 diabetes increases the risk of snoring and, more seriously, breathing difficulties associated with sleep apnea. These problems can ruin the sleep of men and their partners. People with type 1 diabetes can be awakened in the middle of the night by their continuous glucose-monitoring systems, which set off alarms when their blood sugar drops too low. In addition, chronic fatigue syndrome and fibromyalgia are often associated with poor sleep quality and outright insomnia.

Aging   Older people often say they need less sleep, but do they really? Or are their shorter sleep hours reflective of underlying biochemical abnormalities related to general senescence? My hunch is the latter, mainly because advancing age involves a deterioration in the activity of all tissues, hormones, and biochemical processes. Seniors often do not consume sufficient protein, which contains amino acids and vitamins to produce neurotransmitters and other brain chemicals. Low levels of vitamin B_6 alone will inhibit dreaming.

How to Improve Your Sleep Naturally

There are many natural and safe ways to improve sleep. Some involve changes in dietary habits, modification of evening habits, or using natural substances to safely optimize your brain chemistry.

I do not recommend taking prescription drugs to induce sleep. They are part of a lucrative $24 billion sleep business that rarely addresses the causes of poor sleep habits. Ambien, Lunesta, and Sonata treat a symptom—insomnia—and trazodone and benzodiazepines reduce the anxiety that keeps some people awake at night, but all of these drugs do not address the actual cause of sleep problems. Then there are the side effects, such as Ambien users who walk in their sleep and gorge themselves on food or Lunesta users who experience nightmares. These drugs can be addictive or, at the very least, create a dependency (sort of like "addiction lite"). As is the case with any drug, higher doses are eventually needed to achieve the same dubious benefits.

Cut back on caffeine.   It seems like a no-brainer, but excess caffeine consumption is one of the leading causes of poor sleep quality. If you want a better night's sleep, it's essential that you reduce, if not eliminate, all caffeine from your diet.

The most obvious sources of caffeine are coffee, tea, energy drinks, soft drinks, and 5-Hour Energy shots (and variations sold by a variety of companies). Yet some caffeine-containing foods may surprise you. Decaffeinated coffee still retains about 5 percent of its original caffeine content. Chocolate has caffeine in it. So do any chocolate-containing breakfast cereals, such as Kellogg's Cocoa Krispies or Malt-O-Meal. In fact, any product made with chocolate, such as soymilk and many flavored artificial creamers, contains some caffeine.

Many people do fine with one or two cups of coffee in the morning. Yet drinking more than that or consuming caffeinated beverages in the afternoon or the evening increases the odds of their having sleep problems. It's really very simple. If you overstimulate your body (your central nervous system, specifically) during the day, you'll have problems turning it off at night.

Prepare yourself for sleep.   For many people—maybe even for you—going to sleep is not as simple as putting on pajamas and turning off the lights. It would help if you prepared to go to bed and to sleep. Begin by dimming the lights about an hour or so before bedtime. Turn off the television, and don't check your e-mail, make late-night calls, or send texts. As much fun as these activities might be, they tend to stimulate, rather than relax. In fact, the light of your computer monitor may be brighter (given your close proximity) than other lights in a room. Watching a high-intensity action movie isn't conducive to resting. Instead, listen to soft music and read a book or a magazine. Go to bed at a reasonable time—when you are likely to get a full eight hours of sleep. Drink a glass of water about 30 minutes before bedtime, but go to the bathroom to void right before getting into bed. You can keep a glass or a bottle of water next to the bed, but sip it only if you get thirsty during the night. If you live with another person, do your best to avoid arguments before bedtime and do not argue in the bedroom. (As a general rule, always express your disagreements in other rooms.)

Prepare your bedroom for sleep.   Treat your bedroom as if it were a sacred space. This room is for sleep, cuddling, pillow talk, and sex—not for watching television, using a computer or a cell phone, or reading. If you keep a phone in the bedroom, turn off the ringer. Try not to overfurnish the bedroom, and don't use the room (including the space under the mattress) for storage. Make sure you have a comfortable mattress and pillow and that the bedroom is not too warm—a slightly cool room is best for sleep. In addition, minimize your exposure to light, which may mean removing all but the dimmest night lights and getting thick drapes to block ambient light from outside. If you use an alarm clock, turn its face away from you. Even though your eyelids might be closed, your brain will still register all of these lights. If you wake up in the middle of the night, you really don't need to know what time it is and how many hours you have left before the alarm rings.

Consider Natural Sleep Aids

Several dietary supplements can help promote restful sleep.

Melatonin   Melatonin is a hormone that makes us sleepy. Most health food stores and pharmacies sell it. It's safe and might even reduce your risk of getting cancer, although taking too much will leave you feeling groggy the next day. It may take some experimenting to determine the ideal dose for you. Some people respond to very tiny amounts, whereas others need substantially more. Beneficial dosages range from 250 mcg to 3 mg (3,000 mcg). Start with the lowest amount, and increase it each night until you achieve the desired effect. If you take only one tablet, do so about an hour before bedtime. If you take two or more tablets, take the first around dusk to mimic the body's secretion of the hormone and then take more one hour before going to bed.

L-tryptophan and 5-hydroxytryptophan　L-tryptophan and 5-hydroxytryptophan (5-HTP) are the immediate precursors to serotonin, a relaxing and antidepressant neurotransmitter. You can take 50 to 100 mg of 5-HTP, or 500 mg of L-tryptophan, about one hour before bedtime. Either supplement may be of particular benefit if you also suffer from depression.

Gamma amino butyric acid　Gamma amino butyric acid (GABA) is both an amino acid and a neurotransmitter, and L-theanine has neurotransmitter-like effects. Both increase the brain's alpha waves, which are associated with improved mental focus and a sense of relaxation. GABA helps the brain filter out distractions. L-theanine is found in high-quality green tea. Consider taking 200 to 500 mg of GABA and 100 to 200 mg of L-theanine, separately or in combination, about one hour before you go to bed. I like Carlson Laboratories' Mellow Mood (800–323–4141, carlsonlabs.com), which contains GABA, L-theanine, and B vitamins. Other companies sell L-theanine as a standalone supplement.

Magnesium　If your muscles feel tense at bedtime, or if you suffer from restless legs syndrome, either magnesium or vitamin E supplements may bring relief. Muscle spasms (including charley horses) and tightness almost always suggest inadequate magnesium levels. Consider taking 400 mg daily of magnesium citrate or magnesium citrate malate, with meals. If you develop loose stools, divide the dosage so that you take it twice daily, or reduce it slightly.

Valerian   This herb (Valeriana officinalis) has a sedative effect and may be particularly useful if a "busy mind" keeps you from sleeping. Because products vary, follow label directions. *Note:* Do not combine valerian with any other sedative herb, melatonin, tranquilizers, or sleeping pills without checking with a physician or an herbalist who is familiar with herbal remedies.

Should You Take Naps?

Many societies have traditionally allowed for naps after lunch. One could argue that naps are a sign of prediabetic post-meal rises in blood sugar, but one could also make the argument that animals, including people, were not meant to be active for sixteen straight hours.

If you feel like taking a fifteen-minute nap after lunch—and your work allows you to do so—go ahead. There's a good chance that you will have greater energy levels for the rest of the afternoon and be far more productive than you would be otherwise. If you suffer from adrenal burnout or are recovering from it, taking a short nap before 3 p.m. will also likely enhance your energy levels.

The timing and length of a nap are crucial in determining whether your overnight sleep will be affected. If you take a long nap late in the afternoon or early in the evening, you may have difficulty falling asleep when you go to bed. You'll have to do some experimenting to determine what kind of nap energizes you without disrupting your sleep.

In the next and final chapter of *No More Fatigue*, I discuss how light physical activity can improve your energy levels and can even help you get a good night's sleep.

chapter 11

Physical Activity to Boost Your Energy

If you are suffering from the Fatigue Syndrome, by definition you feel tired much of the time. You probably can't imagine exercising—and making yourself even more tired. If you're busy, odds are that you will shake your head and say that you just cannot make room in your schedule to exercise. Your arguments aside, physical activity will increase your energy and stamina, and you don't have to do a lot to reap the benefits.

I offer this advice not as an exercise fanatic or a gym rat. Until 2003, I had been pretty much a lifelong couch potato. I told people I didn't have the time or energy to exercise, and I trusted that my eating habits and supplements would make up for a lack of physical activity. When I finally did begin to exercise, at the urging of a friend, I almost gave up on the first day. I cycled behind her on my first hill, and at the top my lungs and heart were pounding, and I almost vomited. It was not a pretty picture. Yet after a few weeks, my stamina increased and I stopped feeling tired in the afternoon. A year later, in the shower, I happened to notice that my legs had become rock hard. If I can do it, you can do it.

It's important to recognize that all five circles of fatigue can interfere with your need for physical activity. It's hard to imagine making the time for physical activity when you're stressed and already have plenty on your "to do" list. Poor eating habits and low hormone levels can sap your strength and stamina. Chronic illness and age also affect your ability to be active physically.

A Reassurance to Couch Potatoes

Don't worry—I don't plan to act like a drill sergeant, and I won't push you to your physical limits. In fact, as a general rule, I try to avoid using the "E" word, mainly because the word *exercise* has so many negative connotations. It's not merely a matter of conjuring up the energy or the time to exercise. Sometimes we are embarrassed to show our weak or out-of-shape bodies in public at a gym, especially in front of younger people who are really buff.

When I coach people, I try to emphasize physical activity, which is usually less structured and can be a lot more fun than exercise per se. I realize that you are most likely out of shape, so my wish is to encourage you to move, rather than discourage you. My activity recommendations in this chapter follow a graduated regimen that starts very slowly and easily. I won't ask too much of you and, just as important, I don't want you to demand or expect too much of yourself too quickly. Yet it is essential to engage in some type of physical activity every day. This "go easy" suggestion applies doubly if you have osteoarthritis of the knees, patellofemoral (knee cap) pain, or any other serious health problems.

How Physical Activity Revs Up Your Cells

A number of cellular and physiological changes start to occur after you increase your physical activity. First, activity turns on genes that are involved in making muscle and burning fat. Second, your body starts to produce more muscle cells in the area that is doing the work, such as your arms, legs, and heart. Third, new and old muscle cells increase the numbers and the size of mitochondria, the parts of cells that are responsible for breaking down food molecules for energy. In addition, your lung function improves, so that you can take in more air and are more efficient in exhaling as well.

There are many side benefits to the increase in muscle cells and mitochondria. Your body will become much more efficient at burning off fat and lowering your blood sugar, total cholesterol, low-density lipoprotein (LDL) cholesterol, and triglyceride levels. In contrast, drugs such as statins and metformin do nothing more than correct some of the symptoms—chiefly, hypercholesterolemia and hyperglycemia, which result from a lack of physical activity.

Your Reward: A Better-Looking Body and Numerous Health Benefits

There are so many health benefits from regular physical activity. Your risk of heart disease decreases significantly. So does your chance of developing cancer or becoming depressed. One recent study, published in the *British Medical Journal*, found that slow walkers were almost 50 percent more likely than fast walkers to die from cardiovascular disease. It wasn't that slow walking was dangerous, but that walking speed was a marker of overall cardiovascular health. This doesn't mean you should immediately start walking as fast as you can, but rather that you set a goal of increasing your walking speed over several weeks or months.

It's certainly easier to maintain a healthy weight if you are physically active, and that's essential because overweight is a major risk factor for type 2 diabetes, heart disease, and cancer—diseases that can compromise your energy levels. For most people, exercise will burn some calories but, in itself, will not lead to significant weight loss. More important, regular exercise will increase your metabolic rate, so that you burn more calories even when you're sitting or sleeping. To lose substantial amounts of weight—more than just a few pounds—you'll have to combine my dietary recommendations with increased physical activity.

Many people express frustration when they gain weight after adopting an exercise regimen. The explanation for this apparent paradox should offer some reassurance: muscle weighs more than fat. So the real question becomes one of choosing between ten more pounds of muscle or ten less pounds of fat. Given the choice, adding muscle is more important than losing fat. In practical terms, it means paying less attention to your weight on the bathroom scale and more attention to your body proportions and your fat/muscle ratio. You don't have to be obsessive about any of this. You can use a tape measure to check your waist circumference or simply pay attention to whether your jeans or pants are looser.

Two recent studies have particular relevance. Researchers at the University of Alabama, Birmingham, found that men and women who continued to exercise, even after modest increases in weight, did not gain any visceral fat. Visceral fat is intertwined with the organs in your midsection (usually indicated by a big belly), and it is the type of fat that predisposes a person to diabetes and heart disease. Meanwhile, researchers at the University of Colorado, Denver, found that exercise reduced the desire to overeat and curbed the growth of new fat cells when people did regain some weight.

Physical activity is good for your mood as well. Doctors have long known that physical activity can resolve depression and anxiety, but until recently, they did not understand why. It turns out that physical activity prompts the creation of new brain cells, a process called neurogenesis. It also restructures the brain in subtle ways that make brain cells more capable of resisting stress.

Not surprisingly, activity increases your life expectancy. A 2009 study in the journal *Medicine and Science in Sports and Exercise* found that even the lightest forms of physical activity reduced the chances of dying at any age. Furthermore, the lower risk of death and improved longevity aren't only because people are less likely to die from obesity, diabetes, or heart disease. Physical activity boosts the body's production of a particular chemical, nicotinamide phosphoribosyltransferase (NAMPT), which plays a crucial role in activating the SIRT1 gene. This particular gene appears to be the key longevity gene in most species, including humans.

Physical Activity for Everyone

As I have watched many of my older, long-term colleagues in both medicine and the natural foods industry enter their sixties and seventies, I
couldn't help but notice a serious decline in their health. I certainly
expected them to maintain superior health in their later years. Yet many
of these people have focused only on supplements or eating habits, not
on physical activity. One key feature of aging, especially after age seventy, is an increase in physical frailty, weakness, and muscle fatigue. Of
course, there are numerous causes of this frailty, including, as I previously noted, a lack of vitamin D and protein. Because we all lose muscle
mass with age, advancing age really demands that we stay physically
active to maintain as much muscle as possible. We may not be able to
regain the body of a twenty-year-old, but we can develop a fairly good
body for whatever our age happens to be.

It's important to note that my recommendations for physical activity
don't apply only to people who simply feel tired. Regular activity is indispensable for people with serious diseases, such as chronic fatigue syndrome (CFS), fibromyalgia, and cancer. One step for recovering from
CFS is maintaining a regular regimen of physical activity, but beginning very slowly and tailoring the exercise to one's physical tolerance.
Recently, Dutch researchers reported that supervised exercise therapy
reduced knee pain and led to improved physical functioning in people with patellofemoral (knee) pain syndrome. Danish researchers also
showed that regular exercise reduced fatigue and increased vitality, muscular strength, physical functioning, and emotional well-being among
men and women who were undergoing chemotherapy.

A Little Activity Takes Just a Little Effort

The more physical activity or exercise you do on a regular basis, the
greater the benefits—short of seriously overexerting yourself and developing overuse injuries. Yet considerable research has demonstrated that
light activity provides many of the health benefits of more intense activity. One study found that several short and very intense bursts of activity,

adding up to all of six minutes a week, led to increases in endurance almost equal to that of people who exercised at a steady pace for a couple of hours. Those short bursts of energy, however, required people to approach their exercise and pain threshold. I normally don't make the "no pain, no gain" argument, but this seems to be an exception.

As a general rule, maintaining physical fitness requires somewhere between thirty and sixty minutes of physical activity on most days of the week. You can do the same activity or vary the activities; you can be active thirty minutes a day or one hour every other day. You might consider alternating between walking, riding a bicycle (stationary or outdoors), swimming, or using hand weights. The details are your choice. Light but regular physical activity, however, such as going for a stroll, has been shown to improve people's energy levels by about 20 percent. Light workouts, such as regularly using a stationary bicycle, reduced fatigue by 65 percent, according to one study. For most people, combining these activities with dietary improvements and nutritional supplements will lead to a complete recovery from the Fatigue Syndrome.

Keep It Simple—Just Go for a Walk

Some exercise enthusiasts make things too complicated for the average person, such as with specialized and expensive equipment. I almost always suggest walking to people who have not exercised or engaged in any type of regular physical activity. It's easy to pace yourself, and you don't need any special equipment—other than a comfortable pair of shoes.

Motivation Taking that first step is often the most difficult, partly because physical activity is often perceived to be boring. I go for a very brisk walk on the days that I don't cycle, and, while I alternate my route, I do make mental notes of what's the same and what has changed. For example, the pickup truck with the paint splatters is almost always in a certain driveway, and once a week some of the lawns get mowed.

To avoid boredom, it helps to walk with another person. Conversation is a great distraction, although you should always pay attention to where you step to prevent tripping. If you have a dog, you have little choice but to take it out for a walk, but you may need to walk as much as the dog. Another option is to use an MP3 player (such as an iPod) to listen to music. My selection of rock 'n' roll music on my MP3 player keeps my speed up. Other times, I just want to listen to the wheels of my bike spin or to the sound of a breeze, so relative silence often helps me process thoughts, problem solve, or create a meditative state.

Making the time   Until I started a program of regular physical activity, I always wondered how I would find the time in my busy schedule. Physical activity has to be a priority, and I make time for it nearly every day. Sometimes I have to try to work faster or harder to make up for the exercise time, but it's a small price to pay. You can also save time by cutting out some nonphysical activities, such as surfing television channels. In fact, a study in the *Archives of Internal Medicine* found that watching less television led to more physical activity. You can always record the show for later viewing.

Location   Safety is important, so pick a safe location and time of day if you're going for long walks outdoors. Many health centers (such as the YMCA) have indoor tracks for walking and jogging. You can also walk in an indoor shopping mall, which is a particularly good choice when the weather is inclement. Just don't window shop until you finish your workout walk. You can also build walking into shorter "sprints," such as by parking farther from the door or taking the stairs instead of the elevator. Walking down, rather than up, appears to use muscles that do a better job of burning blood sugar, so you might consider taking an elevator up several stories and then walking down the stairs.

Time of day   The hour of the day that you choose to exercise can influence the quality of your workout, and there's growing evidence that exercising in the late afternoon or early evening is ideal for many people. Many people feel a little stiff in the morning. The cause isn't always arthritis but instead a slightly lower body temperature. As the body warms up and you begin to do some simple activities, such as showering and drying, your body temperature increases and your muscles start to limber up. One measure of cardiovascular fitness is being able to achieve a relatively high heart rate, and some research now indicates that a higher heart rate is more easily achieved in the afternoon than in the morning.

Graduated regimen   It is very important that you start walking (or any other type of physical activity) at a slow, easy pace. Do what's comfortable, whether it is a five-minute or a sixty-minute walk. Don't try to overdo, because you will be more likely to either tire or injure yourself. If you're out of shape—this could apply whether you're skinny or fat, young or old—start with a five- to ten-minute walk, such as to the end of your block, simply to see how you respond. As each week goes by, try to increase your distance or speed. Maybe there's an interesting historical part of town for you to walk through and explore. When I travel for book signings or lectures, I often walk long distances—what I call urban hiking.

Other Easy Physical Activities to Do at Home

Stretching may not by itself enhance your energy levels, but it can help you limber up and reduce back pain or spine compression. When you stretch your hamstring, a thigh muscle, you will also stretch your lower back.

Simple Stretches

Stretch 1   Lie on your back on the floor with your legs straight for about 30 seconds. Raise one knee to your chest or as close to your chest as possible, and hold it there for about 15 seconds. It may help to clasp your hands over your shin to bring your knee a couple of inches closer to your chest. Then slowly raise your leg, while keeping it as straight as possible, so that the bottom of your foot points roughly to the ceiling. Hold this position for 15 seconds, then bring your leg down so that it is again straight on the floor. Repeat with your other leg. *Note*: At first, you may have difficulty stretching your leg straight up, but bringing it to a forty-five-degree angle is a good start.

Stretch 2   Sit on the floor and straighten one leg, such as your left. Bend the other leg so that your ankle rests against or near your groin. If you have difficulty, do the best you can. Slowly lower your torso over the straight leg. Try to hold this position for 20 seconds or so. Repeat while bending the other leg. *Note*: If you are right-handed, odds are that your right leg will also be more flexible, so start by keeping your left leg straight and bending your right leg.

Stretch 3   Stand straight, with your arms at your sides and your knees bent slightly. Take a deep breath. Exhale while bending your body forward at your waist. Allow your fingers to touch your toes or the floor or as close as you can get. Hold this position for 20 to 30 seconds. Slowly straighten out and inhale. Repeat two more times.

Simple Training and Toning

With nothing more than a chair and a couple of handweights (3 to 5 pounds each), you can do a number of simple training and toning exercises in the privacy of your home.

Biceps curl   Stand straight up. Have your arms at your sides, hands facing your thighs, holding the weights firmly in each hand. Slowly lift your hands and turn your arms so that the weights face your chest. Slowly bring your arms back so that your hands and the weights are next to your thighs. Repeat five to ten times.

Upper arm presses   Stand straight up, arms bent slightly at your elbows, with the weights in your hands and the weights (and closed palms of your hands) facing forward. Lift the weights slowly above your head, keeping the weights facing forward (away from your body). Slowly lower the weights to shoulder level and then to your starting position. Repeat five to ten times.

> ### *quick tip*
> ### Physical Activity Enhances Sleep Quality
>
> Being more physically active can help you get a better night's sleep. Research with both adults and children has found that daytime physical activity and nighttime sleep are closely related to each other. In one study, every hour of sedentary behavior increased the time it took to fall asleep by about three minutes. If you fall asleep faster, with less tossing and turning, you'll get more sleep.

Upper body toner   Sit on the edge of an armless chair, with your back straight and your feet flat on the floor. Hold the weights on the top of your thighs, palms down. Raise your elbows to shoulder height, bending them to the sides, and hold the weights in front of you, palms facing down. Keep this position for a couple of seconds, then lower your arms and the weights to your starting position.

Do You Need a Recovery Drink or Food?

Other than having a glass of water, you will not need any kind of recovery fluid or food after being physically active for 15 to 30 minutes. If you are very active for at least an hour, such as cycling or very brisk walking, you can consider drinking a recovery fluid or eating some food. Beware, however, of the many recovery drinks and foods that contain too much sugar and are very expensive as well.

If you feel tired after 30 minutes or less of activity, sit in a chair and rest comfortably for a few minutes to recover. My favorite recovery beverage is coconut water, and my preferred brands are Zico (www.zico .com) and O.N.E. (www.onenaturalexperience.com). Coconut water (not coconut milk) is rich in potassium and also contains a very small amount of sodium. This is enough to replace the electrolytes (minerals that are needed to regulate your heartbeat) that you may have lost in sweat. If you develop or have previously experienced charley horses (painful muscle spasms in the lower legs), you should consider the possibility that you are magnesium-deficient. In that case, try taking 200 to

400 mg of magnesium citrate, which you'll find in the supplement section of a natural foods store or pharmacy.

Unless you engage in vigorous exercise for more than an hour, you're also not likely to need any type of energy bar or similar food product. A small amount of protein, such as a couple of bites of chicken, or a piece of fruit should be sufficient.

Do You Need to Carb Load?

Many endurance athletes make a habit of carb loading—that is, consuming a large amount of carbohydrates the night before a marathon or a long bicycle ride. The idea behind carb loading is to increase the liver's reserves of glycogen, a form of stored sugar. The glycogen is typically released when there is a need, such as to prevent hypoglycemia.

If you are engaged in moderate physical activity, you do not have to carb load the night before. In fact, the basic theory behind carb loading is not scientifically sound, and it's often merely an excuse to overeat. The liver normally stores about one to two hours' worth of glycogen, and this amount cannot be significantly increased. Carb loading can create a prediabetic state, however, at least temporarily, that may reduce energy levels.

Loren Cordain, Ph.D., the author of *The Paleo Diet* and *The Paleo Diet Cookbook*, recommends against carb loading because of its effect on blood sugar and energy levels. Instead, he suggests providing nutritional support during the recovery period, specifically a little protein and fruit. Again, this should not be a concern unless you are exercising vigorously for more than one hour.

What about Overuse Injuries?

The postexercise muscle soreness or "burn" has long been attributed to a buildup of lactic acid in muscle tissue. Although many professional and amateur athletes still believe that lactic acid is a cause of muscle soreness, the idea is now scientifically passé. It turns out that lactic acid is actually a cellular fuel, not a cause of soreness. The soreness results from microscopic tears in muscle tissue that trigger a painful inflammatory response.

Weekend warriors—occasional athletes who tend to overdo—are most likely to injure themselves because they are out of shape. Yet even elite athletes experience overuse injuries. In 2001, while I was researching *The Inflammation Syndrome*, I realized that it was relatively easy to use certain nutritional supplements to modulate the inflammatory response. I found that the physical therapist for the Danish Olympic team and several other people in Denmark were thinking along the same lines, but they had an opportunity to put the theory into practice.

Up to that time, Søren Mavrogenis, the Danish physical therapist, had suggested that elite athletes with overuse injuries take over-the-counter analgesics (such as ibuprofen) and rest for a month while healing. The athletes were unhappy about the mandated rest because they would lose much of their training. Mavrogenis began to give the athletes natural anti-inflammatories: omega-3 fish oils, gamma-linolenic acid (a plant oil), and small amounts of antioxidant vitamins. The benefit was significant: pain from the inflammatory overuse injuries decreased, and the athletes were able to continue training.

As I've written, if you begin your physical activity regimen slowly and are careful not to overexert yourself, you are unlikely to experience an overuse injury. If you do, however, I recommend taking Carlson Laboratories' Inflammation Balance supplement (carlsonlabs.com), which is similar to the supplement given to Danish athletes.

It is so easy not to engage in regular physical activity—sometimes we're short on time, other times we're just plain lazy. Yet the health benefits of moderate activity are simply too great for us to ignore. Being active is as important as good nutrition, water, and supplements. Comparing my couch potato days to my current level of regular activity, I now understand what so many people had told me for years: being active increases energy levels.

Afterword

Making changes in one's life can be a scary proposition. After all, we're creatures of habit, and change means getting used to doing things a little differently. Sometimes the known, as unpleasant as it might be, feels much more comfortable than the unknown.

Yet there are times when we must make those changes—to create better health, improve our energy levels, and alter the lifestyle habits that led to our Fatigue Syndrome.

No one should lack the energy he or she needs to enjoy a full and satisfying life. Yet millions of people barely muster up the strength to begin and get through each day. No one should live with feelings of being totally stressed out. Yet millions suffer from tension and pressures that drain their energy each and every day. Stress and fatigue often go hand in hand, and they force many people to depend on an assortment of stimulants to keep going.

Think back for a moment. When you were a child, your energy was effortless and practically boundless. You played, you learned, you wanted to do everything, and you practically did. Yet somewhere along the way toward adulthood, your energy levels started to diminish. You became more dependent on stimulants of one sort or another, such as caffeine and sugar.

Of all of the recommendations I've made in this book, breaking or at least lessening the grip of the caffeine habit may be the most difficult. For many people, the thought of not having coffee or an energy drink can be terrifying, especially if your work and home life stretch you to the limit, and you need caffeine to give you that extra push. That situation alone could be a sign of adrenal exhaustion, which I discussed in chapter 3.

As I've written, however, both caffeine and sugar are actually anti-energy foods. They may provide a brief boost, but they set you up for a drop in your energy level.

I'm sure you understand it intellectually, but the unease of changing your habit or the fear of not having caffeine may very well be holding you back. That's the power of a food addiction, which can be just as strong as a drug or alcohol addiction.

Having said that, I am a realist and a pragmatist, and I understand the dilemma you face. I know that you might not be able to completely eliminate caffeine and sugar.

So I'll take this opportunity to remind you of my advice.

1. Caffeine and sugar cannot replace the energy-enhancing and energy-sustaining benefits of a wholesome diet, one that starts with eating a protein-centered breakfast.
2. Caffeine and sugar create a roller-coaster effect on your energy levels. To maintain steady energy throughout the day, you have to rely on protein and high-fiber vegetables and some of the nutritional supplements I've recommended, such as coenzyme Q10 and L-carnitine.
3. A significant dependence on caffeine—for example, more than a couple cups of coffee in the morning—may be a sign of low adrenal or thyroid hormone levels. I believe that both of these hormone problems are far more common than most physicians

realize. If you're drinking more than five cups of coffee daily or find yourself needing coffee in the afternoon or the evening, it's worth asking your physician to run some tests to assess your adrenal and thyroid function.

4. If you simply cannot imagine ever giving up caffeine and sugar, at least work toward reducing your intake of them. Trust me, you can brew weaker coffee or dilute it with Teecchino (teecchino .com), a tasty coffee substitute sold at many health food stores.

Early in the book, I referred to Dr. Albert Szent-Györgyi's idea, based on biochemistry and biology, that energy was the "currency" of life. The truth is that your energy and mine are finite, much like our savings and investments. If the economic recession of 2009 and 2010 taught us anything, it was about the importance of saving money. The same guiding principle applies to preserving energy as well.

To live well, with the health and vitality we all want, it's essential that we manage our personal energy resources as best as we can. It does us no good to waste our energy or to invest in junk foods, the way many people invested in junk bonds. It's much better to preserve and judiciously use our energy. It is my wish that you have the energy to enjoy every day of your life.

Resources for Supplements, Foods, and Additional Information

Nutrition Coaching

Author and nutrition expert Jack Challem is available for individualized nutrition coaching sessions in person in Tucson, Arizona, or by telephone with anyone in the world. For more information and a downloadable brochure, please visit www.jackchallem.com or www.cureyourfatigue. com. For fees and to arrange a coaching appointment, e-mail Jack at jchallem@aol.com.

Nutritionally Oriented Physicians

Nutritionally oriented physicians tend to have a solid understanding of the role of nutrition and biochemistry in illness and generally emphasize nonpharmaceutical therapies. The following organizations can provide the names and qualifications of their physician members, either via their Web sites or by e-mail. Do note that most of these physicians work in a traditional fee-for-service manner, and that insurance companies may not cover any or all of their treatments.

International Society for Orthomolecular Medicine
www.orthomed.org or centre@orthomed.org
American College for Advancement in Medicine
www.acam.org
American Association of Naturopathic Physicians
www.naturopathic.org
The Riordan Clinic
Nutritionally (Biochemically) Oriented Medical Center
3100 N. Hillside Avenue
Wichita, KS 67219
(316) 682-3100

My Newsletter and Books

My newsletter and some of my previous books can provide you with in-depth information on a variety of topics that I briefly discussed in *No More Fatigue*. The books are available from the publisher (www.wiley .com) and from booksellers.

The Nutrition Reporter
> Jack Challem's monthly newsletter summarizes recent research on vitamins, minerals, and herbs. The annual subscription rate is $28 (for Canadian subscribers, $34 U.S. or $40 CND; for all other countries, $42 U.S.). Sample issues in PDF format are available for free at nutritionreporter.com. For a hard-copy sample issue, send a business-size self-addressed envelope, with postage for 2 ounces, to: The Nutrition Reporter, P.O. Box 30246, Tucson, AZ 85751.

The Inflammation Syndrome (Hoboken, NJ: John Wiley & Sons, 2010)
> The 2003 edition of this groundbreaking book described how inflammatory diseases were related to one another and could be resolved through improved nutrition and supplements. This

updated and revised edition provides the latest research on anti-inflammation nutritional supplements.

Stop Prediabetes Now (Hoboken, NJ: John Wiley & Sons, 2007)

This book focuses on the intertwined health problems of overweight and prediabetes. These two conditions stimulate inflammation through a variety of mechanisms. The book includes dietary and supplement guidelines for losing weight and improving blood sugar.

The Food-Mood Solution (Hoboken, NJ: John Wiley & Sons, 2007)

This book explains how food and individual nutrients can prevent or bring about bad moods, such as irritability, anger, anxiety, impulsiveness, and depression. It includes dietary tips and supplement recommendations.

Feed Your Genes Right (Hoboken, NJ: John Wiley & Sons, 2005)

This book focuses on how our genes depend on vitamins and other nutrients and how we can make the most of our genetic inheritance and reduce the risk of disease.

Sources of High-Quality Nutritional Supplements

Thousands of companies sell proprietary brands of vitamins, minerals, and other types of nutritional supplements. I've found the following companies to have good-quality, reliable products.

Carlson Laboratories

Carlson Laboratories makes Nutra-Support Energy: Natural Fatigue Fight supplements—as the names suggest, this formula contains nutrients involved in cellular energy production. The company also makes Nutra-Support Diabetes, a high-potency multivitamin/multimineral supplement formulated specifically for the nutritional needs of people with prediabetes and diabetes. The company is well known for its fish oil supplements, including a lemon-flavored cod liver oil; the widest selection of natural vitamin E products; and a complete assortment of other vitamin and mineral supplements. For more information, call (800) 323-4141 or go to www.carlsonlabs.com.

Nutricology/Allergy Research Group

Nutricology/Allergy Research Group is often at the cutting edge of original nutritional supplement formulations. Nutricology is the company's consumer brand, and Allergy Research Group is the company's professional (physician's) brand. For more information, call (800) 545-9960 or go to www.nutricology .com.

Solgar Vitamin and Herb

This company markets an extensive line of vitamin, mineral, and herb supplements, which are sold in the United States, Europe, and most other regions of the world. I've known Dr. Richard Passwater, the company's director of research, for more than thirty years, and I have always been impressed with his knowledge and formulations. For more information, go to www .solgar.com.

Terry Naturally

This company markets many beneficial products, including a high-potency curcumin supplement (CuraMed), a plant-based anti-inflammatory formula (Curacel), and many other fine products. For more information, visit www.europharmausa.com. Like many of the other brands listed here, Terry Naturally is also sold at health and natural food stores.

Natural Food Grocers

I recommend that you eat nutrient-dense fresh and natural foods. Your best bet for finding meat from range- or grass-fed animals and organic fruits and vegetables is at a natural foods or specialty grocery store. Many cities have locally owned natural food markets. The three I list here have a national or strong regional presence.

Natural Grocers by Vitamin Cottage

Formerly known simply as Vitamin Cottage, this family-owned chain of stores sells organic foods and has one of the largest retail selections of nutritional supplements. It currently has approximately thirty stores, most of them in Colorado, but also some in New Mexico, Texas, and Utah. The owners are among the most ethical business people I've met, and one of the things I really like about Vitamin Cottage is its commitment to education with free public lectures. You can order products online or search for store locations at www.vitamincottage.com.

Trader Joe's

Trader Joe's is a chain of high-quality specialty retail grocery stores, with many organic, gluten-free, and wholesome products. It's not a health food market, though, and it's always important to read the list of ingredients on packaged foods. For more information and the locations of Trader Joe's stores, go to www .traderjoes.com.

Whole Foods

Whole Foods is the largest chain of natural food markets in the United States. The emphasis is on wholesome and organic foods. The quality is high, and, unfortunately, the prices tend to be as well. Whether you're in Whole Foods or other natural food markets, it is important to always read the ingredients list on any packaged food. Unnecessary sugars and carbs are often added. For more information, go to www.wholefoodsmarket.com.

Distinctive Food Products

Eden Foods

Eden is a well-established natural food company that sells its products through natural food stores. Most of the products are also available by mail order. In chapter 8, I recommend two specific pasta substitutes sold by Eden. One is Kuzu Pasta, which is gluten-free and derived from the root of a plant. It has a similar jellylike texture (think of it as a fun food) to that of Japanese shirataki noodles. The other Eden product I recommend is Buckwheat Soba, which is made in Japan from 100 percent buckwheat—an herb, not a grain. (Most buckwheat soba noodles are a blend of whole wheat and buckwheat.) Because the Buckwheat Soba is processed in a facility that also handles wheat, Eden cannot guarantee that it is gluten-free, but odds are that it is. For more information, go to www.edenfoods.com.

Lotus Foods (Exotic Rice)

Lotus Foods sells a variety of original and tasty rice and rice flour products, including Bhutanese Red Rice and purple Forbidden Rice. The rice flours can be used to dredge fish and chicken, as well as to make gluten-free crepes. For more information, call (510) 525-3137 or go to www.lotusfoods.com to order or find recipes.

MacNut Oil (Macadamia Nut Oil)

MacNut Oil, made from Australian macadamia nuts, is rich in oleic acid, the same type of fat that makes olive oil so healthy. MacNut Oil has a slightly nutty flavor and a higher smoke point than olive oil. For information, call (866) 462-2688 or go to www .macnutoil.com.

Miroku (Green Tea)

I tried for years to find a good-quality green tea that I could brew as an iced tea. They all tasted weak. Then I found "Catechin-Rich Tea" in a Japanese grocery store in San Francisco. It's organically grown, and each tea bag makes an entire pitcher of tea, which brews within about fifteen minutes on your kitchen countertop. It has a rich flavor, and I drink it with nearly all of my meals. You can order it online from Miroku by visiting www .miroku-usa.com.

Olivado (Avocado Oil)

Avocado oil is rich in anti-inflammatory oleic acid (an omega-9 fat). It has a high smoke point and a neutral flavor that doesn't dominate foods the way that some types of olive oil do. The marketer of these oils, Olivado, sells pure cold-pressed avocado oil and several varieties of avocado oil infused with basil, lemon, rosemary, or chili. These oils have amazing subtleties and can be used both in cooking and as oil-and-vinegar salad dressings. For more information, go to www.olivado.com.

The Spice House

I recently discovered the Spice House, with its four stores in the Chicago area and a mail order business. Most of the Spice House's herbs and spices are sold in bulk, although a few are bottled for the convenience of customers. The Spice house has several curry blends—remember, curry contains many potent anti-inflammatory ingredients. The "hot" curry powder is traditional and spicy, although you can control its hotness by using less or more in recipes. If you want the benefits of curry without any of the heat, try the Spice House's "sweet" curry powder. It's not sweet; it simply doesn't have any hot pepper in the blend. The employees are very helpful. For more information, visit www.thespicehouse.com or call (847) 328-3711.

Coconut Water

Several companies now market coconut water in 11-ounce containers. I think the best brands are O.N.E., Zico, and Harvest Bay. For more information, visit www.onenaturalexperience.com, www.zico.com, nakedjuice.com, and www.harvest-bay.com.

Helpful Web Sites

Medline/PubMed

The world's largest searchable database of medical journal articles, providing free abstracts (summaries) of more than 8 million articles. www.pubmed.gov

Nutrient Data Laboratory Food Composition

Type in nearly any food or food product, and you instantly get its nutritional breakdown per cup or 100 grams. www.nal.usda.gov/fnic/foodcomp

Making a Self-Diagnosis

Two Web sites can help you sort through your symptoms and make an initial self-diagnosis, which may help you before you see a physician. One is www.wrongdiagnosis.com. The other is www .merck.com/mmpe/index.html, where you will find the online edition of the Merck Manual, which is a physician's reference. You can search both for free, but do remember that physicians have much more rigorous training in making diagnoses. These sites can head you in the right direction, but you may still need to see a specialist for a precise diagnosis.

Understanding Laboratory Tests

For many people, a copy of their blood tests is nearly impossible to interpret. This Web site is one of the best for explaining what the tests mean: www.aruplab.com/.

Yoga for Depression

Amy Weintraub cured her own depression through yoga, and, as the founder of LifeForce Yoga, she has helped thousands of people work through their own mood issues. Amy has a rare gift as a teacher. You can order a copy of her book *Yoga for Depression*, buy copies of her CDs, subscribe to her free online newsletter, and learn about her workshops at her Web site: www .yogafordepression.com.

References

Introduction

Hartman Group. HartBeat In-Depth: Energy Drinks, accessed August 22, 2007, www .hartman-group.com/products/HB/indepth/2007_08_22energy.php.

Puetz, T. W., Flowers, S. S., O'Connor, P. J. A randomized controlled trial of the effect of aerobic exercise training on feelings of energy and fatigue in sedentary young adults with persistent fatigue. *Psychotherapy and Psychosomatics* 77 (2008): 167–174.

1 Stress and Fatigue

Arnedt, J. T., Owens, J., Crouch, M., Stahl, J., and Carskadon, M. A. Neurobehavioral performance of residents after heavy night call vs after alcohol ingestion. *Journal of the American Medical Association* 294 (2005): 1025–1033.

Brackbill, R. M., Hadler, J. L., DiGrande, L., et al. Asthma and posttraumatic stress symptoms 5 to 6 years following exposure to the World Trade Center terrorist attack. *Journal of the American Medical Association* 302 (2009): 502–516.

Cohen, D. L., Wintering, N., Tolles, V., et al. Cerebral blood flow effects of yoga training: Preliminary evaluation of 4 cases. *Journal of Alternative and Complementary Medicine* 15 (2009): 9–14.

Erdmann, J., Kallabis, B., Oppel, U., et al. Development of hyperinsulinemia and insulin resistance during the early stage of weight gain. *American Journal of Physiology, Endocrinology, and Metabolism* 294 (2008): E568–E575.

Henig, R. M. Driving? Maybe you shouldn't be reading this. *New York Times*, July 13, 2005, p. D5.

Hoge, C. W., Castro, C. A., Messer, S. C., et al. Combat duty in Iraq and Afghanistan, mental health problems, and barriers to care. *New England Journal of Medicine* 351 (2004): 13–22.

Horowitz, S. Effect of positive emotions on health. *Alternative and Complementary Therapies* 15 (2009): 196–202.

Ophir, E., Nass, C., and Agner, A. D. Cognitive control in media multitaskers. *Proceedings of the National Academy of Sciences* (2009): doi 10.1073/pnas.0903620106.

Tubelius, P., Stan, V., and Zachrisson, A. Increasing work-place healthiness with the probiotic Lactobacillus reuteri: A randomized, double-blind placebo-controlled study. *Environmental Health: A Global Access Science Source* 4, no. 25 (2005): doi 10.1186/1476–069X-4-25.

Weintraub, A. *Yoga for Depression: A Compassionate Guide to Relieve Suffering through Yoga.* New York: Broadway Books, 2004.

2   Eating Habits and Fatigue

Anderson, C., and Horne, J. A. A high sugar content, low caffeine drink does not alleviate sleepiness but may worsen it. *Human Psychopharmacology* 21 (2006): 299–303.

Arble, D. M., Bass, J., Laposky, A. D., et al. Circadian timing of food intake contributes to weight gain. *Obesity* (Silver Spring) 17 (2009): 2100–2102.

Ataka, S., Tanaka, M., Nozaki, S., et al. Effects of oral administration of caffeine and D-ribose on mental fatigue. *Nutrition* 24 (2008): 233–238.

Bischoff-Ferrari, H. A., Orav, E. J., and Dawson-Hughes, B. Effect of cholecalciferol plus calcium on falling in ambulatory older men and women. *Archives of Internal Medicine* 166 (2006): 424–430.

Burdakov, D., Lensen, L. T., Alexopoulos, H., et al. Tandem-pore K+ channels mediate inhibition of orexin neurons by glucose. *Neuron* 50 (2006): 711–722.

Chiu, K. C., Chu, A., Go, V. L., et al. Hypovitaminosis D is associated with insulin resistance and beta-cell dysfunction. *American Journal of Clinical Nutrition* 79 (2004): 820–825.

Clauson, K. A., Shields, K. M., McQueen, C. E., et al. Safety issues associated with commercially available energy drinks. *Journal of the American Pharmacists Association* 48 (2008): e55–e63.

Cornelis, M. C., El-Sohemy, A., Kabagambe, E. K., et al. Coffee, CYP1A2 genotype, and risk of myocardial infarction. *Journal of the American Medical Association* 295 (2006): 1135–1141.

Croezen, S., Visscher, T. L. S., Ter Bogt, N. C. W., et al. Skipping breakfast, alcohol consumption and physical inactivity as risk factors for overweight and obesity in adolescents: Results of the E-MOVO project. *European Journal of Clinical Nutrition* 63 (2009): 405–412.

Flicker, L., MacInnis, R. J., Stein, M. S., et al. Should older people in residential care receive vitamin D to prevent falls? Results of a randomized trial. *Journal of the American Geriatric Society* 53 (2005): 1881–1888.

Johnston, C. S., Corte, C., and Swan, P. D. Marginal vitamin C status is associated with reduced fat oxidation during submaximal exercise in young adults. *Nutrition & Metabolism* 3 (2006): 35.

Krohn, J., Taylor, F. A., Larson, E. M. *The Whole Way to Allergy Relief & Prevention.* Point Roberts, WA: Hartley & Marks, 1991, pp. 77–78.

Léone, J., Delhinger, V., Maes, D., et al. Rheumatic manifestations of scurvy. A report of two cases. *Revue du Rhumatisme* (English ed.) 64 (1997): 428–431.

Levine, M., Conry-Cantilena, C., Wang, Y., et al. Vitamin C pharmacokinetics in healthy volunteers: Evidence for a recommended dietary allowance. *Proceedings of the National Academy of Sciences* 93 (1996): 3704–3709.

Liu, P. T., Stenger, S., Li, H., et al. Toll-like receptor triggering of a vitamin D-mediated human antimicrobial response. *Science* 311 (2006): 1770–1773.

Packer, C. D. Cola-induced hypokalaemia: A super-sized problem. *International Journal of Clinical Practice* 63 (2009): 833–835.

Pittas, A. G., Harris, S. S., Stark, P. C., et al. The effects of calcium and vitamin D supplementation on blood glucose and markers of inflammation in nondiabetic adults. *Diabetes Care* 30 (2007): 980–986.

Pittas, A. G., Lau, J., Hu, F. B., et al. The role of vitamin D and calcium in type 2 diabetes. A systematic review and meta-analysis. *Journal of Clinical Endocrinology and Metabolism* 92 (2007): 2017–2029.

Purslow, L. R., Sandhy, M. S., Forouhi, N., et al. Energy intake at breakfast and weight change: Prospective study of 6,764 middle-aged men and women. *American Journal of Epidemiology* 167 (2007): 188–192.

Roehrs, T., and Roth, T. Caffeine: Sleep and daytime sleepiness. *Sleep Medicine Reviews* 12, no. 2 (April 2008): 153–162.

Ross, G. W., Abbott, R. D., Petrovitch, H., et al. Association of coffee and caffeine intake with the risk of Parkinson disease. *Journal of the American Medical Association* 283 (2000): 2674–2679.

Shults, C. W., Oakes, D., Kieburtz, K., et al. Effects of coenzyme Q10 in early Parkinson disease. Evidence of slowing of the functional decline. *Archives of Neurology* 59 (2002): 1541–1550.

Szent-Györgyi, A. V. On vitamins, health and disease. In *On Oxidation, Fermentation, Vitamins, Health and Disease*. Baltimore, MD: Williams & Wilkins, 1939, pp. 88–109.

Timlin, M. T., Pereira, M. A., Story, M., et al. Breakfast eating and weight change in a 5-year prospective analysis of adolescents: Project EAT (Eating Among Teens). *Pediatrics* 121 (2008): e638–e645.

Tsimihodimos, V., Kakaidi, V., and Eilisaf, M. Cola-induced hypokalaemia: Pathophysiological mechanisms and clinical implications. *International Journal of Clinical Practice* 63 (2009): 900–902.

Van Dam, R. M., and Hu, F. B. Coffee consumption and risk of type 2 diabetes. *Journal of the American Medical Association* 294 (2005): 97–104.

Vander Wal, J. S., Marth, J. M., Khosla, P., et al. Short-term effect of eggs on satiety in overweight and obese subjects. *Journal of the American College of Nutrition* 24 (2005): 510–515.

Yeom, H. H., Jung, G. C., Shin, S. W., et al. Changes in worker fatigue after vitamin C administration. *Journal of Orthomolecular Medicine* 23 (2008): 205–209.

Zasloff, M. Fighting infections with vitamin D. *Nature Medicine* 12 (2006): 388–390.

3 Hormones and Fatigue

Anonymous. Diagnosis and treatment of adrenal dysfunction. Q & A with James L. Wilson, N.D., D.C., Ph.D. *Focus* (Allergy Research Group Newsletter) (March 2008): 7–9.

Bunevicius, R., Kazanavicius, G., Zalinkevicius, R., et al. Effects of thyroxine as compared with thyroxine plus triiodothyronine in patients with hypothyroidism. *New England Journal of Medicine* 340 (1999): 424–429.

Combs, G. F., Midthune, D. N., Patterson, K. Y., et al. Effects of selenomethionine supplementation on selenium status and thyroid hormone concentrations in healthy adults. *American Journal of Clinical Nutrition* 89 (2009): 1808–1814.

Davis, S. R., Moreau, M., Kroll, R., et al. Testosterone for low libido in postmenopausal women not taking estrogen. *New England Journal of Medicine* 359 (2008): 2005–2017.

Fox, C. S., Pencina, M. J., D'Agostino, R. B., et al. Relations of thyroid function to body weight. *Archives of Internal Medicine* 168 (2008): 587–592.

Oelkers, W. Dehydroepiandrosterone for adrenal insufficiency. *New England Journal of Medicine* 341 (1999): 1073–1074.

Santini, F., Chiovato, L., Rocchi, R., et al. Influences of thyroid diseases in diabetic pregnant women. *Annali dell'Istituto superiore di sanita* 33 (1997): 441–445.

Smithson, M. J. Screening for thyroid dysfunction in a community population of diabetic patients. *Diabetic Medicine* 15 (1998): 148–150.

Van Uum, S. H. Liquorice and hypertension. *Netherlands Journal of Medicine* 63 (2005): 119–120.

Weiss, R. E., and Brown, R. L. Doctor . . . Could it be my thyroid? *Archives of Internal Medicine* 168 (2008): 568–569.

Wilson, J. L. *Adrenal Fatigue: The 21st Century Stress Syndrome*. Petaluma, CA: Smart Publications, 2001.

4 Illness and Fatigue

Atamna, H., Newberry, J., Erlitzki, R., Schultz, C. S., and Ames, B. N. Biotin deficiency inhibits heme synthesis and impairs mitochondria in human lung fibroblasts. *Journal of Nutrition* 137 (2007): 25–30.

Arvold, D. S., Odean, M. J., Dornfeld, M. P., et al. Correlation of symptoms with vitamin D deficiency and symptom response to cholecalciferol treatment: A randomized controlled trial. *Endocrinology Practice* 15 (2009): 203–212.

Baker, S. K., and Tarnopolsky, M. A. Statin myopathies: Pathophysiologic and clinical perspectives. *Clinical and Investigative Medicine* 24 (2001): 258–272. [Note chart on p. 261.]

Bartley, J. Prevalence of vitamin D deficiency among patients attending multidisciplinary tertiary pain clinic. *New Zealand Medical Journal* 121 (2008): 57–62.

Berman, M., Erman, A., Ben-Gal, T., et al. Coenzyme Q10 in patients with end-stage heart failure awaiting cardiac transplantation: A randomized, placebo-controlled study. *Clinical Cardiology* 27 (2004): 295–299.

Blee, T. H., Cogbill, T. H., and Lambert P. J. Hemorrhage associated with vitamin C deficiency in surgical patients. *Surgery* 131 (2000): 408–412.

Block, K. I., Koch, A. C., Mead, M. N., et al. Impact of antioxidant supplementation on chemotherapeutic efficacy: A systematic review of the evidence from randomized controlled trials. *Cancer Treatment Reviews* 33 (2007): 407–418.

Borsheim, E., Bui, Q. U. T., Tissier, S., et al. Effect of amino acid supplementation on muscle mass, strength and physical function in elderly. *Clinical Nutrition* 27, no. 2 (2008): 189–195.

Burns, C. P., Halabi, S., Clamon, G., et al. Phase II study of high-dose fish oil capsules for patients with cancer-related cachexia. *Cancer* 101 (2004): 370–378.

Chiu, G. Vitamin D deficiency among patients attending a central New Zealand rheumatology outpatient clinic. *New Zealand Medical Journal* 118 (2005): U1727.

Cho, H. J., Seeman, T. E., Bower, J. E., et al. Prospective association between C-reactive protein and fatigue in the coronary artery risk development in young adults study. *Biological Psychiatry* 66 (2009): 871–878.

Cordero, M. D., Moreno-Fernández, A. M., deMiguel, M., et al. Coenzyme Q10 distribution in blood is altered in patients with fibromyalgia. *Clinical Biochemistry* 42 (2009): 732–735.

Davis, J. M., Murphy, E. A., Carmichael, M. D., et al. Quercetin increases brain and muscle mitochondrial biogenesis and exercise tolerance. *American Journal of Physiology: Regulatory, Integrative, and Comparative Physiology* 296, no. 4 (2009): R1071–R1077.

Depeint, F., Bruce, W. R., Shangari, N., et al. Mitochondrial function and toxicity: Role of the B vitamin family on mitochondrial energy metabolism. *Chemico-Biological Interactions* 163 (2006): 94–112.

Drisko, J. A., Chapman, J., and Hunter, V. J. The use of antioxidants with first-line chemotherapy in two cases of ovarian cancer. *Journal of the American College of Nutrition* 22 (2003): 118–123.

Duconge, J., Miranda-Massari, J. R., González, M. J., et al. Vitamin C pharmacokinetics after continuous infusion in a patient with prostate cancer. *Annals of Pharmacotherapy* 41 (2007): 1082–1083.

Duconge, J., Miranda-Massari, J. R., Gonzalez, M. J., et al. Pharmacokinetics of vitamin C: Insights into the oral and intravenous administration of ascorbate. *Puerto Rico Health Sciences Journal* 27 (2008): 7–19.

Escrich, E., Moral, R., Grau, L., et al. Molecular mechanisms of the effects of olive oil and other dietary lipids on cancer. *Molecular Nutrition and Food Research* 51 (2007): 1279–1292.

Fiorani, M., Guidarelli, A., Blasa, M., et al. Mitochondria accumulate large amounts of quercetin: Prevention of mitochondrial damage and release upon oxidation of the extramitochondrial fraction of the flavonoid. *Journal of Nutritional Biochemistry* (2009): epub ahead of print.

Gamignano, G., Lusso, M. R., Madeddu, C., et al. Efficacy of L-carnitine administration on fatigue, nutritional status, oxidative stress, and related quality of life in 12 advanced cancer patients undergoing anticancer therapy. *Nutrition* 22 (2006): 136–145.

Giuseppe, C., Elisa, F., Claudio, L., and Maria, R. A. Cadmium and mitochondria. *Mitochondrion* (2009): epub ahead of print.

Heim, C., Nater, U. M., Maloney, E., et al. Childhood trauma and risk for chronic fatigue syndrome: Association with neuroendocrine dysfunction. *Archives of General Psychiatry* 72 (2009): 72–80.

Jurna, I. Analgesic and analgesia-potentiating action of B vitamins. *Schmerz* 12 (1998): 136–141.

Jurna, I., and Reeh, P. W. How useful is the combination of B vitamins and analgesic agents? *Schmerz* 6 (1992): 224–226.

Lee, P., and Chen, R. Vitamin D as an analgesic for patients with type 2 diabetes and neuropathic pain. *Archives of Internal Medicine* 168 (2008): 771–772.

Jitomir, J., and Willoughby, D. S. Leucine for retention of lean mass on a hypocaloric diet. *Journal of Medicinal Food* 11 (2008): 606–609.

Khokhar, J. S., Brett, A. S., and Desai, A. Vitamin D deficiency masquerading as metastatic cancer: A case series. *American Journal of the Medical Sciences* 337 (2009): 245–247.

Kira, J., Tobimatsu, S., and Goto, I. Vitamin B12 metabolism and massive-dose methyl vitamin B12 therapy in Japanese patients with multiple sclerosis. *Internal Medicine* 33 (1994): 82–86.

Konat, G. W., Kraszpulski, M., James, I., et al. Cognitive dysfunction induced by chronic administration of common cancer chemotherapeutics in rats. *Metabolic Brain Disease* 23 (2008): 325–333.Langsjoen, P. H., Vadhanavikit, S., and Folkers, K. Effective treatment with coenzyme Q10 of patients with chronic myocardial disease. *Drugs Under Experimental and Clinical Research* 11 (1985): 577–579.

—— Response of patients in classes III and IV of cardiomyopathy to therapy in a blind and crossover trial with coenzyme Q10. *Proceedings of the National Academy of Sciences of the USA* 82 (1985): 4240–4244.

Langsjoen, P. H., and Langsjoen, A. M. The clinical use of HMG CoA-reductase inhibitors and the associated depletion of coenzyme Q10. A review of animal and human publications. *BioFactors* 18 (2003): 101–111.

Laviano, A., Meguid, M. M., Preziosa, I., et al. Oxidative stress and wasting in cancer. *Current Opinion in Clinical Nutrition and Metabolic Care* 10 (2007): 449–456.

Lebrun, C., Alchaar, H., Candito, M., et al. Levocarnitine administration in multiple sclerosis patients with immunosuppressive therapy-induced fatigue. *Multiple Sclerosis* 12 (2006): 321–324.

Lee, P., Nair, P., Eisman, J. A., et al. Vitamin D deficiency in the intensive care unit: An invisible accomplice to morbidity and mortality? *Intensive Care Medicine* (2009): epub ahead of print.

Lister, R. E. An open, pilot study to evaluate the potential benefits of coenzyme Q10 combined with Ginkgo biloba extract in fibromyalgia syndrome. *Journal of International Medical Research* 30 (2002): 195–199.

Liu, P. T., Stenger, S., Li, H., et al. Toll-like receptor triggering of a vitamin D-mediated human antimicrobial response. *Science* 311 (2006): 1770–1773.

Lockwood, K., Moesgaard, S., and Folkers, K. Partial and complete regression of breast cancer in patients in relation to dosage of coenzyme Q10. *Biochemical and Biophysical Research Communications* 199 (1994): 1504–1508.

Lockwood, K., Moesgaard, S., Yamamoto, T., and Folkers, K. Progress on therapy of breast cancer with vitamin Q10 and the regression of metastases. *Biochemical and Biophysical Research Communications* 212 (1995): 172–177.

Lombardi, V. C., Ruscetti, F. W., Das Gupta, J., et al. Detection of an infectious retrovirus, XMRV, in blood cells of patients with chronic fatigue syndrome. *Science* (2009): epub ahead of print.

Martin, D. P., Sletten, C. D., Williams, B. A., et al. Improvement in fibromyalgia symptoms with acupuncture: Results of a randomized controlled trial. *Mayo Clinic Proceedings* 81 (2006): 749–757.

Medina-Santillan, R., Perez-Flores, E., Mateos-Garcia, E., et al. A B-vitamin mixture reduces the requirements of diclofenac after tonsillectomy: A double-blind study. *Drug Development Research* 66 (2006): 36–39.

Mohaupt, M. G., Karas, R. H., Babiychuk, E. B., et al. Association between statin-associated myopathy and skeletal muscle damage. *Canadian Medical Association Journal* 181 (2009): E11–E18.

Moss, R. W. Do antioxidants interfere with radiation therapy for cancer? *Integrative Cancer Therapies* 6 (2007): 281–292.

Nathens, A. B, Neff, M. J., Jurkovich, G. J., et al. Randomized, prospective trial of antioxidant supplementation in critically ill surgical patients. *Annals of Surgery* 236 (2002): 814–822.

Op den Kamp, C. M., Langen, R. C., Haegens, A., et al. Muscle atrophy in cachexia: Can dietary protein tip the balance? *Current Opinion in Clinical Nutrition and Metabolic Care* (2009): epub ahead of print.

Padayatty, S. J., Riordan, H. D., Hewitt, S. M., et al. Intravenously administered vitamin C as cancer therapy: Three cases. *Canadian Medical Association Journal* 174 (2006): 937–942.

Perumal, S. S., Shanthi, P., and Sachdanandam, P. Energy-modulating vitamins—a new combinatorial therapy prevents cancer cachexia in rat mammary carcinoma. *British Journal of Nutrition* 93 (2005): 901–909.

Plioplys, A. V., and Plioplys, S. Amantadine and L-carnitine treatment of chronic fatigue syndrome. *Neuropsychobiology* 35 (1997): 16–23.

Pradhan, A. D., Everett, B. M., Cook, N. R., et al. Effects of initiating insulin and metformin on glycemic control and inflammatory biomarkers among patients with type 2 diabetes. *Journal of the American Medical Association* 302 (2009): 1186–1194.

Premkumar, V. G., Yuvaraj, S., Vijayasarathy, K., et al. Effect of coenzyme Q10, riboflavin and niacin on serum CEA and CA 15–3 levels in breast cancer patients undergoing tamoxifen therapy. *Biological and Pharmaceutical Bulletin* 30 (2007): 367–370.

Rao, C. V., Newmark, H. L., and Reddy, B. S. Chemopreventive effect of squalene on colon cancer. *Carcinogenesis* 19 (1998): 287–290.

Reynolds, E. H., Linnell, J. C., and Faludy, J. E. Multiple sclerosis associated with vitamin B12 deficiency. *Archives of Neurology* 48 (1991): 808–811.

Rossini, M., Di Munno, O., Valentini, G., et al. Double-blind, multicenter trial comparing acetyl l-carnitine with placebo in the treatment of fibromyalgia patients. *Clinical and Experimental Rheumatology* 25 (2007): 182–188.

Rumelin, A., Humbert, T., Luhker, O., et al. Metabolic clearance and the antioxidant ascorbic acid in surgical patients. *Journal of Surgical Research* 129 (2005): 46–51.

Seppa, N. Patients deficient in vitamin D fare worse in battle with lymphoma. *Science News* (web edition), accessed December 5, 2009, www.sciencenews.org/view/generic/id/50452/title/Patients_deficient_in_vitamin_D_fare_worse_in_battle_with_lymphoma.

Siddiqui, R., Pandya, D., Harvey, K., et al. Nutrition modulation of cachexia/proteolysis. *Nutrition in Clinical Practice* 21 (2006): 155–167.

Silver, M. A., Langsjoen, P. H., Szabo, S., et al. Effect of atorvastatin on left ventricular diastolic function and ability of coenzyme Q10 to reverse that dysfunction. *American Journal of Cardiology* 94 (2004): 1306–1310.

Simone, C. B., 2nd, Simone, N. L., Simone, V., et al. Antioxidants and other nutrients do not interfere with chemotherapy or radiation therapy and can increase kill and increase survival, part 1. *Alternative Therapies in Health and Medicine* 13 (2007): 22–28.

———. Antioxidants and other nutrients do not interfere with chemotherapy or radiation therapy and can increase kill and increase survival, part 2. *Alternative Therapies in Health and Medicine* 13 (2007): 40–47.

Solerte, S. B., Gazzaruso, C., Bonacasa, R., et al. Nutritional supplements with oral amino acid mixtures increase whole-body lean mass and insulin sensitivity in elderly subjects with sarcopenia. *American Journal of Cardiology* 101, suppl. (2008): 69E–77E.

Sotiroudis, T. G., and Kyrtopoulos, S. A. Anticarcinogenic compounds of olive oil and related biomarkers. *European Journal of Nutrition* 47, suppl. 2 (2008): 69–72.

Sugino, T., Shirai, T., Kajimoto, Y., et al. L-ornithine supplementation attenuates physical fatigue in healthy volunteers by modulating lipid and amino acid metabolism. *Nutrition Research* 28 (2008): 738–743.

Tomassini, V., Pozzilli, C., Onesti, E., et al. Comparison of the effects of acetyl L-carnitine and amantadine for the treatment of fatigue in multiple sclerosis: Results of a pilot, randomised, double-blind, crossover trial. *Journal of the Neurological Sciences* 218 (2004): 103–108.

Waterman, E., and Lockwood, B. Active components and clinical applications of olive oil. *Alternative Medicine Review* 12 (2007): 331–342.

Yeom, C. H., Jung, G. C., and Song, K. J. Changes of terminal cancer patients' health-related quality of life after high dose vitamin C administration. *Journal of Korean Medical Science* 22 (2007): 7–11.

Zasloff, M. Fighting infections with vitamin D. *Nature Medicine* 12 (2006): 388–390.

5 Aging and Fatigue

Blount, B. C., Mack, M. M., Wehr, C. M., et al. Folate deficiency causes uracil misincorporation into human DNA and chromosome breakage: Implications for cancer and neuronal damage. *Proceedings of the National Academy of Sciences* 94 (1997): 3290–3295.

Chan, R., Woo, J., Suen, E., et al. Chinese tea consumption is associated with longer telomere length in elderly Chinese men. *British Journal of Nutrition* (2009): epub ahead of print.

Christensen, K. Thinggaard, M., McGue, M., et al. Perceived age as clinically useful biomarker of ageing: Cohort study. *British Medical Journal* 339 (2009): b5262.

Everson, R. B., Mehr, C. M., Erexson, G. L., et al. Association of marginal folate depletion with increased human chromosomal damage in vivo: Demonstration by analysis
of micronucleated erythrocytes. *Journal of the National Cancer Institute* 80 (1988):
525–529.

Fenech, M., Aitken, C., and Rinaldi, J. Folate, vitamin B12, homocysteine status and
DNA damage in young Australian adults. *Carcinogenesis* 19 (1998): 1163–1171.

Harman, D. The free radical theory of aging. *Antioxidants and Redox Signaling* 5
(2003): 557–561.

———. Role of free radicals in aging and disease. *Annals of the New York Academy of Science* 673 (1992): 126–141.

Killilea, D. W., and Ames, B. N. Magnesium deficiency accelerating cellular senescence in cultured human fibroblasts. *Proceedings of the National Academy of
Sciences* 105 (2008): 5768–5773.

Oltean, S., and Banerjee, R. Nutritional modulation of gene expression and homocysteine utilization by vitamin B12. *Journal of Biological Chemistry* 278 (2003):
20778–20784.

Rossi, E. L. Sacred spaces and places in healing dreams: Gene expression and brain
growth in rehabilitation. *Psychological Perspectives* 47 (2004): 48–63.

Spronck, J. C., Batleman, A. P., Boyonoski, A. C., et al. Chronic DNA damage and niacin
deficiency enhance cell injury and cause unusual interactions in NAD and Poly(ADP-
ribose) metabolism in rat bone marrow. *Nutrition and Cancer* 45 (2003): 124–131.

6 Supplements to Jump-Start Your Energy

Ames, B. N., Elson Schwab, H., and Silver, E. A. High-dose vitamin therapy stimulates
variant enzymes with decreased coenzyme binding affinity (increased Km): Relevance to genetic disease and polymorphisms. *American Journal of Clinical Nutrition*
75 (2002): 616–658.

Ames, B. N. Low micronutrient intake may accelerate the degenerative diseases of aging
through allocation of scarce micronutrients by triage. *Proceedings of the National
Academy of Sciences of the USA* 103 (2006): 17589–17594.

Barbiroli, B., Medori, R., Tritschler, H. J., et al. Lipoic (thioctic) acid increases brain
energy availability and skeletal muscle performance as shown by in vivo 31P-MRS in
a patient with mitochondrial cytopathy. *Journal of Neurology* 242 (1995): 472–477.

Belardinelli, R., Mucaj, A., Lacalaprice, F., et al. Coenzyme Q10 improves contrac-
tility of dysfunctional myocardium in chronic heart failure. *Biofactors* 25 (2005):
137–145.

Belardinelli, R., Mucaj, A., Lacalaprice, F., et al. Coenzyme Q10 and exercise training
in chronic heart failure. *European Heart Journal* 27, no. 22 (2006): 2675–2681.

Berman, M., Erman, A., Ben-Gal, T., et al. Coenzyme Q10 in patients with end-stage
heart failure awaiting cardiac transplantation: A randomized, placebo-controlled
study. *Clinical Cardiology* 27 (2004): 295–299.

Borsheim, E., Bui, Q. U., Tissier, S., et al. Effect of amino acid supplementation on
muscle mass, strength and physical function in elderly. *Clinical Nutrition* 27, no. 2
(2008): 189–195.

Bronstein, A. C., Spyker, D. A., Cantilena, J. R., et al. 2007 Annual Report of the American Association of Poison Control Centers' National Poison Data System (NPDS): 25th Annual Report. *Clinical Toxicology* 46 (2008): 927–1057. Download at www.aapcc.org/DNN/Portals/0/NPDS%20reports/2008%20AAPCC%20Annual%20Report.pdf.

Cooke, M., Iosia, M., Buford, T., et al. Effects of acute and 14-day coenzyme Q10 supplementation on exercise performance in both trained and untrained individuals. *Journal of the International Society of Sports Nutrition* 5 (2008): 8.

Davis, J. M., Murphy, E. A., McClellan, J. L., et al. Quercetin reduces susceptibility to influenza infection following stressful exercise. *American Journal of Physiology—Regulatory, Integrative and Comparative Physiology* 295 (2008): R505–R509.

Davis, J. M., Murphy, E. A., and Carmichael, M. D. Effects of the dietary flavonoid quercetin upon performance and health. *Current Sports Medicine Reports* 8 (2009): 206–213.

Davis, J. M., Murphy, E. A., Carmichael, M. D., et al. Quercetin increases brain and muscle mitochondrial biogenesis and exercise tolerance. *American Journal of Physiology—Regulatory, Integrative and Comparative Physiology* 296 (2009): R1071–R1077.

Elmadfa, I., Majchrzak, D., Rust, P., et al. The thiamine status of adult humans depends on carbohydrate intake. *International Journal for Vitamin and Nutrition Research* 71 (2001): 217–221.

McCann, J. C., and Ames, B. N. Vitamin K, an example of triage theory: Is micronutrient inadequacy linked to diseases of aging? *American Journal of Clinical Nutrition* 90 (2009): 889–907.

Folkers, K., and Simonsen, R. Two successful double-blind trials with coenzyme Q10 (vitamin Q10) on muscular dystrophies and neurogenic atrophies. *Biochimica et Biophysica Acta* 1271 (1995): 281–286.

Hagen, T. M., Liu, J., Lykkesfeldt, J., et al. Feeding acetyl-L-carnitine and lipoic acid to old rats significantly improves metabolic function while decreasing oxidative stress. *Proceedings of the National Academy of Sciences of the USA* 99 (2002): 1870–1875.

Jitomir, J., and Willoughby, D. S. Leucine for retention of lean mass on a hypocaloric diet. *Journal of Medicinal Food* 11 (2008): 606–609.

Koopman, R., Verdijk, L., Manders, R. J., et al. Co-ingestion of protein and leucine stimulates muscle protein synthesis rates to the same extent in young and elderly lean men. *American Journal of Clinical Nutrition* 84 (2006): 623–632.

Langsjoen, P. H., and Langsjoen, A. M. The clinical use of HMG CoA-reductase inhibitors and the associated depletion of coenzyme Q10. A review of animal and human publications. *BioFactors* 18 (2003): 101–111.

Langsjoen, P. H., Langsjoen, A., Willis, R. A., et al. The aging heart: Reversal of diastolic dysfunction in the elderly with oral coenzyme Q10. In *Anti-Aging Medical Therapeutics*, R. M. Klatz and R. Goldman, eds. Marina del Rey, CA: Health Quest Publications, 1997, pp. 113–120.

Langsjoen, P. H., Langsjoen, J. O., Langsjoen, A. M., and Lucas, L. A. Treatment of statin adverse effects with supplemental coenzyme Q10 and statin drug discontinuation. *BioFactors* 25 (2005): 147–152.

Levine, M., Conry-Cantilena, C., Wang, Y., et al. Vitamin C pharmacokinetics in healthy volunteers: Evidence for a recommended dietary allowance. *Proceedings of the National Academy of Sciences of the USA* 93 (1996): 3704–3709.

Liu, J., Killilea, D. W., and Ames, B. N. Age-associated mitochondrial oxidative decay: Improvement of carnitine acetyltransferase substrate-binding affinity and activity in brain by feeding old rats acetyl-L-carnitine and/or R-a-lipoic acid. *Proceedings of the National Academy of Sciences of the USA* 99 (2002): 1876–1881.

Lockwood, K., Moesgaard, S., Yamamoto, T., et al. Progress on therapy of breast cancer with vitamin Q10 and the regression of metastases. *Biochemical and Biophysical Research Communications* 212 (1995): 172–177.

Malaguarnera, M., et al. L-Carnitine treatment reduces severity of physical and mental fatigue and increases cognitive functions in centenarians: A randomized and controlled clinical trial. *American Journal of Clinical Nutrition* 86 (2007): 1738–1744.

Milgram, N. W., Araujo, J. A., Hagen, T. M., et al. Acetyl-L-carnitine and alpha-lipoic acid supplementation of aged beagle dogs improves learning in two landmark discrimination tests. *FASEB Journal* 21 (2007): 3756–3762.

Mizuno, K., Tanaka, M., Nozaki, S., et al. Antifatigue effects of coenzyme Q10 during physical fatigue. *Nutrition* 24 (2008): 293–299.

Pauling, L. Orthomolecular psychiatry. Varying the concentrations of substances normally present in the human body may control mental disease. *Science* 160 (1968): 265–271.

Sandor, P. S., Clemente, D., Coppola, G., et al. Efficacy of coenzyme Q10 in migraine prophylaxis: A randomized controlled trial. *Neurology* 64 (2005): 713–715.

Shults, C. W., Oakes, D., Kieburtz, K., et al. Effects of coenzyme Q10 in early Parkinson disease. Evidence of slowing of the functional decline. *Archives of Neurology* 59 (2002): 1541–1550.

Solerte, S. B., Gazzaruso, C., Bonacasa, R., et al. Nutritional supplements with oral amino acid mixtures increase whole-body lean mass and insulin sensitivity in elderly subjects with sarcopenia. *American Journal of Cardiology* 101, suppl. (2008): 69E–77E.

Sugino, T., Shirai, T., Kajimoto, Y., et al. L-ornithine supplementation attenuates physical fatigue in healthy volunteers by modulating lipid and amino acid metabolism. *Nutrition Research* 28 (2008): 738–743.

Van Gammerren, D., Falk, D., and Antonio, J. The effects of four weeks of ribose supplementation on body composition and exercise performance in healthy, young, male recreational bodybuilders: A double-blind, placebo-controlled trial. *Current Therapeutic Research—Clinical and Experimental* 63 (2002): 486–495.

7   Eating for Energy

Croezen, S., Visscher, T. L. S., Ter Bogt, N. C. W., et al. Skipping breakfast, alcohol consumption and physical inactivity as risk factors for overweight and obesity in adolescents: Results of the E-MOVO project. *European Journal of Clinical Nutrition* 63, no. 3 (March 2009): 405–412.

Farshchi, H. R., Taylor, M. A., and Macdonald, I. A. Deleterious effects of omitting breakfast on insulin sensitivity and fasting lipid profiles in healthy lean women. *American Journal of Clinical Nutrition* 81 (2005): 388–396.

Liljeberg, H. G. M., Akerberg, A. K. E., and Bjorck, I. M. E. Effect of the glycemic index and content of indigestible carbohydrates of cereal-based breakfast meals on glucose tolerance at lunch in healthy subjects. *American Journal of Clinical Nutrition* 69 (1999): 647–655.

Purslow, L. R., Sandhy, M. S., Forouhi, N., et al. Energy intake at breakfast and weight change: Prospective study of 6,764 middle-aged men and women. *American Journal of Epidemiology* 167 (2007): 188–192.

Timlin, M. T., Pereira, M. A., Story, M., et al. Breakfast eating and weight change in a 5-year prospective analysis of adolescents: Project EAT (Eating Among Teens). *Pediatrics* 121 (2008): e638–e645.

Vander Wal, J. S., Marth, J. M., Khosla, P., et al. Short-term effect of eggs on satiety in overweight and obese subjects. *Journal of the American College of Nutrition* 24 (2005): 510–515.

9 Reducing Stress to Ease Your Fatigue

Brackbill, R. M., Hadler, J. L., DiGrande, L., et al. Asthma and posttraumatic stress symptoms 5 to 6 years following exposure to the World Trade Center terrorist attack. *Journal of the American Medical Association* 302 (2009): 502–516.

Cohen, D. L., Wintering, N., Tolles, V., et al. Cerebral blood flow effects of yoga training: Preliminary evaluation of 4 cases. *Journal of Alternative and Complementary Medicine* 15 (2009): 9–14.

Hoge, C. W., Castro, C. A., Messer, S. C., et al. Combat duty in Iraq and Afghanistan, mental health problems, and barriers to care. *New England Journal of Medicine* 351 (2004): 13–22.

Horowitz, S. Effect of positive emotions on health. *Alternative and Complementary Therapies* 15 (2009): 196–202.

Tubelius, P., Stan, V., and Zachrisson, A. Increasing work-place healthiness with the probiotic Lactobacillus reuteri: A randomized, double-blind placebo-controlled study. *Environmental Health: A Global Access Science Source* 4, no. 25 (2005): doi:10.1186/1476–069X-4-25.

Weintraub, A. *Yoga for Depression: A Compassionate Guide to Relieve Suffering through Yoga*. New York: Broadway Books, 2004.

10 Learning to Sleep Well

Ayas, N. T., White, D. P., Manson, J. E., et al. A prospective study of sleep duration and coronary heart disease in women. *Archives of Internal Medicine* 163 (2003): 205–209.

Saey, T. H. The why of sleep. *Science News* (October 24, 2009): 17–23.

Wertz, A. T, Wright, K. P., Ronda, J. M., et al. Effects of sleep inertia on cognition. *Journal of the American Medical Association* 295 (2006): 163–164.

11 Physical Activity to Boost Your Energy

Adamsen, L., Quist, M., Andersen, C., et al. Effect of a multimodal high intensity exercise intervention in cancer patients undergoing chemotherapy: Randomised controlled trial. *British Medical Journal* 339 (2009): b3410 doi: 10.1136/bmj.b3410.

Brooks, G. A. Lactate doesn't necessarily cause fatigue: Why are we surprised? *Journal of Physiology* 536, part 1 (2001): 1.

Costford, S. R., Bajpeyi, S., Pasarica, M., et al. Skeletal muscle NAMPT is induced by exercise in humans. *American Journal of Physiology, Endocrinology and Metabolism* (2009): epub ahead of print.

Dumurgier, J., Elbaz, A., Ducimetiere, P., et al. Slow walking speed and cardiovascular death in well functioning older adults: Prospective cohort study. *British Medical Journal* 339 (2009): b4460 doi: 10.1136/bmj.b4460.

Hunter, G. R., Chandler-Laney, P. C., Brock, D. W., et al. Fat distribution, aerobic fitness, blood lipids, and insulin sensitivity in African-American and European-American women. *Obesity* (2009): epub ahead of print.

Kolata, G. Lactic acid is not muscles' foe, it's fuel. *New York Times*, May 16, 2006, www.nytimes.com/2006/05/16/health/nutrition/16run.html?_r=1&scp=1&sq=lactic%20acid&st=cse.

―――. Ready to exercise? Check your watch. *New York Times*, December 10, 2009, pp. E1, E10.

MacLean, P. S., Higgins, J. A., Wyatt, H. R., et al. Regular exercise attenuates the metabolic drive to regain weight after long-term weight loss. *American Journal of Physiology—Regulatory, Integrative and Comparative Physiology* 297 (2009): R793–R802.

Mandic, S., Myers, J. N., Oliveira, R. B., et al. Characterizing differences in mortality at the low end of the fitness spectrum. *Medicine & Science in Sports & Exercise* 41 (2009): 1573–1579.

Otten, J. J., Jones, K. E., Littenberg, B., et al. Effects of television viewing reduction on energy intake and expenditure in overweight and obese adults. *Archives of Internal Medicine* 169 (2009): 2109–2115.

Puetz, T. W., Flowers, S. S., and O'Connor, P. J. A randomized controlled trial of the effect of aerobic exercise training on feelings of energy and fatigue in sedentary young adults with persistent fatigue. *Psychotherapy and Psychosomatics* 77 (2008): 167–174.

Van Linschoten, R., Van Middelkoop, M., Berger, M. Y., et al. Supervised exercise therapy versus usual care for patellofemoral pain syndrome: An open label randomised controlled trial. *British Medical Journal* 339 (2009): b4074 doi: 10.1136/bmj.b4074.

Index

About the Author

Jack Challem, known as The Nutrition Reporter, is a personal nutrition coach and one of America's most trusted health writers. He is a member of the American Society for Nutrition and the best-selling author of more than twenty books, including *Stop Prediabetes Now, The Food-Mood Solution, The Inflammation Syndrome, Feed Your Genes Right,* and *Syndrome X*. Jack is a columnist for the journal *Alternative & Complementary Therapies* and serves on the editorial board of the *Journal of Orthomolecular Medicine*. His scientific articles have appeared in *Free Radical Biology & Medicine, Journal of Orthomolecular Medicine, Medical Hypotheses*, and other journals. He writes *The Nutrition Reporter* newsletter as well as articles for many publications in the United States, Canada, and the United Kingdom. Free, downloadable excerpts from his books and sample issues of his newsletter are available at www.nutritionreporter.com.